Welcome to

THE
EVERYTHING
HEALTH GUIDES ®

When you're faced with a pressing health issue, your first instinct is to find out as much about it as you can. With so much conflicting information out there, where can you turn for professional, supportive advice?

Packed with the most recent, up-to-date data, THE EVERYTHING® HEALTH GUIDES help ensure that you get a good diagnosis, choose the best doctor, and find the right medical treatment. With this one comprehensive resource, you and your family members have all the information you could possibly need—at your fingertips.

THE EVERYTHING® HEALTH GUIDES are an extension of the best-selling Everything® series in the health category, which also includes *The Everything® Diabetes Book* and *The Everything® Menopause Book*. Accessible and easy to read, THE EVERYTHING® HEALTH GUIDES provide specific details and clear examples that relate to your given medical situation. If you're looking for one-stop, all-inclusive guides that allow you to understand and become more in tune with your body, this groundbreaking series is the perfect tool for you.

Visit the entire Everything® series at *www.everything.com*

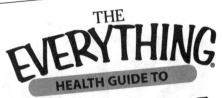

THE EVERYTHING®

HEALTH GUIDE TO

POSTPARTUM CARE

Dear Reader,

After I gave birth to my first child nine years ago, I found myself with a sudden lack of information. While books and frequent prenatal care appointments had walked me through each week of pregnancy, after I was discharged from the hospital I felt like I was on my own. Books detailed the basics of baby care and breastfeeding, but I couldn't find a single source of comprehensive information about what to expect as I recovered from childbirth and adjusted physically and emotionally to my new role as a mother.

After speaking to countless new mothers, I see that the same questions I had come up again and again: Will I ever get enough sleep again? How can I keep my marriage strong? Will I be able to get my old body back? What if I get postpartum depression? Is it normal to feel conflicted about motherhood?

As a new mother, you probably have those questions and more, and *The Everything® Health Guide to Postpartum Care* has the answers. This book addresses the physical, emotional, and practical issues new mothers face, helping you to take good care of yourself, enjoy your baby, and find confidence in yourself as a mother.

Best wishes,

Meagan Francis

THE

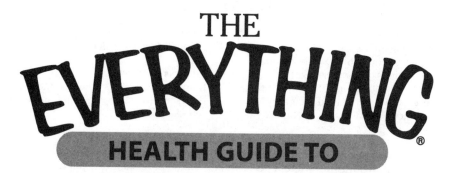

EVERYTHING

HEALTH GUIDE TO

POSTPARTUM CARE

A complete guide to looking and feeling
great after delivery and beyond

Meagan Francis

with Technical Review by Kip Kozlowski, R.N., C.N.M.

Adams Media
Avon, Massachusetts

This book is dedicated to the staff, clients, and founding midwives of the Greenhouse Birth Center.

Publisher: Gary M. Krebs
Managing Editor: Laura M. Daly
Associate Copy Chief: Shelia Zwiebel
Acquisitions Editor: Kerry Smith
Development Editor: katie McDonough
Associate Production Editor: Casey Ebert
Technical Reviewer: Kip Kozlowski

Director of Manufacturing: Susan Beale
Production Project Manager:
Michelle Roy Kelly
Prepress: Erick DaCosta, Matt LeBlanc
Layout and Graphics: Heather Barrett,
Brewster Brownville, Colleen Cunningham,
Jennifer Oliveira

An Everything® Series Book.
Everything® and everything.com® are registered trademarks of F+W Publications, Inc.

Published by Adams Media, an F+W Publications Company
57 Littlefield Street, Avon, MA 02322 U.S.A.
www.adamsmedia.com

ISBN 10: 1-59869-275-5
ISBN 13: 978-1-59869-275-4

Printed in Canada.

J I H G F E D C B A

Library of Congress Cataloging-in-Publication Data
Francis, Meagan.
The everything health guide to postpartum care /
Meagan Francis, with technical review by Kip Kozlowski.
p. cm.—(An everything series book)
ISBN-13: 978-1-59869-275-4 (pbk.)
ISBN-10: 1-59869-275-5 (pbk.)
1. Postnatal care—Popular works. 2. Motherhood—Popular works. 3. Childbirth—Popular
works. 4. Infants—Care—Popular works. I. Title. II. Title: Health guide to postpartum care.

RG801.F73 2007
618.6—dc22
2007001120

This publication is designed to provide accurate and authoritative information with regard to the subject matter covered. It is sold with the understanding that the publisher is not engaged in rendering legal, accounting, or other professional advice. If legal advice or other expert assistance is required, the services of a competent professional person should be sought.
—From a *Declaration of Principles* jointly adopted by a Committee of the
American Bar Association and a Committee of Publishers and Associations

Many of the designations used by manufacturers and sellers to distinguish their products are claimed as trademarks. Where those designations appear in this book and Adams Media was aware of a trademark claim, the designations have been printed with initial capital letters.

This book is available at quantity discounts for bulk purchases.
For information, please call 1-800-289-0963.

*All the examples and dialogues used in this book are fictional and have
been created by the author to illustrate medical situations.*

Acknowledgments

Very special thanks to Kip Kozlowski, R.N., C.N.M., for the wealth of knowledge she contributed to this book. And a big thank you to Clarice Winkler, C.N.M.; Mitzi Montague-Bauer, doula extraordinaire; and Shelie Ross, C.N.M., all of the Greenhouse Birth Center, for answering endless questions, and also for the wise and thorough care they provide women (myself included) before, during, and after birth.

I'd also like to thank the women of YAAPS.com, the GBC moms, my sister Kathreen, and my sister-in-law Jenna for lending so much of their personal experiences to this book—it was immensely helpful.

Endless thanks to my husband, Jon, for his unwavering support, and of course, to my sons Jacob, Isaac, William, and Owen, who gave me firsthand understanding of all things postpartum, from baby elation to sleep deprivation.

And thanks to Gina Panettieri for walking this first-timer through the often-murky waters of book publishing.

Contents

Introduction

In some cultures, a woman who's had a baby is expected to rest for a month or more while the other members of the community or tribe care for her. In the United States, it's more likely that a new mom would be expected back at work within a month or two. New mothers are sent home from the hospital with directions to return to their doctors in six weeks, but myriad emotional and physical issues come up during that time. Unfortunately, many women are left to work through these concerns on their own, or are often unsure of where to look for help when a question comes up.

There is much more to the postpartum period than feeding and diapering. When a baby is born, a mother is born, too, and the changes she experiences can be confusing and unexpected. You'll go through a myriad of physical changes. After birth, your body will begin its shift back to its prepregnancy shape and size. As your organs shift, your uterus shrinks, and your body rids itself of excess fluid, your breasts will begin producing milk, and your hormone levels will fluctuate. As you're going through this major physiological transformation, you'll also be getting to know your little one and, if this is your first baby, adjusting to a whole new set of responsibilities and lifestyle changes that can bring on a huge emotional response.

It's a lot of changing to go through in just a few short months. Yet the postpartum period is often overlooked in books about parenting and motherhood, which tend to focus on the baby's care and development. The same tends to happen in our culture—at birth, the focus shifts from the pregnant woman to her baby, and the result is often that the needs of the postpartum woman are overlooked. And while we think of the postpartum period as being the six weeks after delivery, in reality a new mother will continue to experience hormonal, physical, and emotional postpartum changes for months after she gives birth.

Postpartum can be a wonderful time when women are given the opportunity to slow down, rest, and get to know the new baby they've carried and given birth to. It can also be a stressful time. Adding a new baby can tax the relationship between a mother and father, which can be even more difficult to deal with when nobody's getting enough sleep, and a pile of dirty diapers is stacking up.

The keys to thriving—rather than just surviving—through the postpartum period include having enough help, trusting in your abilities as a mother, taking good care of yourself by eating well and getting as much sleep as possible, and having realistic expectations of yourself, your baby, and your partner. This book will help you do just that. By explaining in detail what you can expect from your physical recovery from birth and how you can navigate your emotional adjustment to new motherhood, including information on diet and nutrition, exercise, wardrobe, postpartum depression, sex, and more, *The Everything® Health Guide to Postpartum Care* will act as your guide to preparing for and blossoming during this exciting and transformational time of your life.

Congratulations on the birth of your new baby! I wish you plenty of support, enough sleep, and much patience as you take the journey through new motherhood.

Preparing for a Great Postpartum Experience

MANY EXPECTING MOMS SPEND a lot of time preparing—shopping, reading, and learning—to care for a baby. This is certainly a necessary part of getting ready for your little one to arrive. But too many moms-to-be forget to make a plan for their own postpartum health and happiness at the same time. Pull together the tools, help, and knowledge you'll need before your baby is born, and you'll be well on your way to having a relaxing and happy postpartum experience.

How Your Birth Experience Affects Your Postpartum Experience

Your birth experience affects so much more than just how and when your baby is born. Every procedure and intervention used during your labor, from medications used to start or augment your labor, to pain medication or anesthesia, to fetal monitoring, IVs, and even the position you're in when you push your baby out, can have an effect on how easily and comfortably you recover after your baby is born.

When making a birth plan, you should take into account not only how interventions and drugs can affect your baby and delivery, but also how they might make you feel postpartum. The following sections cover some common interventions and procedures used during labor, and how they might affect your recovery after giving birth.

Induction

When your labor is induced, it can increase the chances that you'll end up with a long, hard labor, and it makes it more likely that you'll need additional interventions like pain medication, epidural anesthesia, or even a cesarean section. Many care providers induce routinely, and not all have sound medical reasons for doing so.

Narcotic Pain Relief

Drugs like Demerol, Stadol, and Nubain can all cause you to feel spacy and out of it in your baby's first minutes, and can make nursing difficult. And once your baby is born, the drugs can take weeks to leave your system.

Epidurals

Epidurals can lead to a host of side effects, including severe headaches, fever, pain and itching at the site of the injection, uneven numbing, and occasionally, even more severe side effects like a sudden drop in blood pressure. Epidurals make it more likely that you'll have a forceps delivery, episiotomy, birth by c-section, and other interventions that can make recovery more difficult.

Antibiotics

The routine use of antibiotics during labor and birth isn't uncommon, but it can cause postpartum problems. You may have an allergic reaction to an antibiotic, which could mar your postpartum experience with side effects. Also, antibiotics can cause yeast infections by wiping out the healthy bacteria in your system that keep fungi in check. Nursing moms can also get yeast infections of the nipples, called thrush, which can be painful for both mom and baby. Make sure you know whether your care provider intends to give you antibiotics during your labor and birth, under what circumstances, and what alternatives you may have. You may have to do some research on your own to find out this information.

Essential

If you know ahead of time that you'll have antibiotics during labor and birth, eat lots of yogurt containing live bacteria cultures or take acidophilus supplements, which you can find in your health-food store or pharmacy. This will help maintain the balance of micro-organisms in your body and reduce your risk of yeast infection.

Fetal Monitoring

Constant external fetal monitoring can limit your movement or even keep you stuck in bed, which can make it more difficult to deal with contractions and respond to your baby's passage through your body, and can increase the chances that you'll have an epidural or other pain medication.

Alert

There's no scientific evidence that constant fetal monitoring creates better birth outcomes for low-risk mothers having normal preg-nancies, but it may increase the chance of of having a c-section and other interventions. Ask if your provider and birthplace will consider placing you on the monitor only intermittently, or consider using a portable Doppler to check your baby's heartbeat instead of an elec-tronic fetal monitor.

Internal fetal monitoring involves a care provider placing an electrode on your baby's scalp while he is still inside your uterus. Any time hands or objects are in your vagina during labor, you run a higher risk of developing an infection, which can make you very sick postpartum. There's also a risk of infection to your baby's scalp.

Also, care providers must rupture your bag of waters to place the electrodes on your baby's scalp, which further increases your risk of intervention and infection. Sometimes, however, accurate fetal monitoring will prevent an unnecessary c-section, and internal monitoring is much more reliable than external monitoring.

Forceps or Vacuum Extraction

Using forceps or vacuum extraction during your birth can damage your pelvic floor, cause tearing and trauma, and increase both your pain during and after birth and the amount of time it'll take you to heal postpartum.

Episiotomy

An episiotomy is an incision made through layers of tissue and muscle in the perineum. While an episiotomy is usually unnecessary, many care providers do them routinely. They are painful, can take longer to heal than natural tears, and can increase the risk of infection. Ask your health-care provider about his or her episiotomy rates, and how he or she will work with you to help you avoid episiotomies. Giving birth in an upright position, experiencing perineal massage or support while pushing, and pushing when you have the urge (as opposed to forced or "coached" pushing) can all help your baby emerge more easily without an episiotomy.

C-section

Deliveries by cesarean section can be lifesaving when used appropriately, but most experts agree that there are far too many c-sections performed in the United States. If you have your baby via c-section, you can plan on a longer, more painful recovery, increased risk of infection, and a host of other short- and long-term side effects.

If you hope to have a baby vaginally in the future, you'll want to do all you can to avoid an unnecessary c-section this time around. Because of rising malpractice rates and fears of litigation, it's becoming increasingly more difficult to find care providers and hospitals that will allow mothers with previous c-sections to deliver vaginally.

Avoiding Interventions

If you think you'd like to avoid any of the previously discussed interventions during your birth, don't wait and see how things go when you're actually in labor. Instead, arm yourself with knowledge and the intention to have the birth experience you want.

Negative birth experiences have been linked with postpartum depression and even posttraumatic stress disorder. No provider can guarantee that you'll have the outcome you hope for, but giving birth with a provider you really trust and feeling like a partner in your own care can help you understand what happened and give you a feeling of peace about your birth experience, even if it didn't go perfectly according to plan.

Learn All You Can

Read books on childbirth, study comfort techniques, and learn about methods like Lamaze or birth hypnosis. Take a childbirth-education class, but don't be discouraged if the teacher seems to assume you'll end up with a very medical birth—if that's not what you want, you can work toward something different. See Appendix B for a list of resources that can help you educate yourself.

Communicate Your Wishes

By the time you've reached your last trimester of pregnancy, you should be talking with your doctor or midwife about his or her philosophy on birth and intervention, as well as how he or she plans to help you avoid unnecessary and unwanted medications or other procedures. Sooner is better than later here, since you may want to switch providers if you find that your current caregiver is unable or unwilling to assist you in pursuing the kind of birth you want.

Check Out Your Birthplace

The hospital or birth center where you'll give birth will likely have a larger say in what goes on during your labor than your provider, who may not even arrive on the scene until you're ready to push. It's very important to tour the place where you intend to give birth and find out its policies and procedures. Will you be able to eat and drink during labor? What about IVs and routine fetal monitoring? How will they help you with breastfeeding? Not all lactation consultants are created equal.

 Question

How can I know if my hospital or birth center is breastfeeding friendly?

Unicef and the World Health Organization (WHO) have created the Baby-Friendly Hospital Initiative, which gives its stamp of approval to hospitals and birthing centers that follow ten steps to make the facility breastfeeding friendly, such as allowing unrestricted breastfeeding and helping mothers initiate breastfeeding within an hour of birth. Visit *www.babyfriendlyusa.org* for more information.

Hire Help

Consider hiring a doula to assist you with your birth. A doula will provide support in achieving the birth experience you want and act as an advocate on your behalf. She can free your husband or partner up from the stressful job of coach, and make sure your wishes are communicated to the medical staff and that you understand any procedures or interventions your doctor or midwife wants to perform. For more information on finding a birth doula, visit Appendix B.

Communicate Again

Even if your doctor or midwife is very familiar with your birth plan, it's still crucial to inform the nurses on staff when you go into labor. In most hospitals and many birth centers, nurses do the majority of the labor care—as mentioned previously, your doctor may not even arrive until you're ready to push!

Ŀ. Essential

Sometimes, the nurses in a maternity unit will have preferences for the kind of birth (i.e., highly medicated or low intervention) they like best, and will try to match up their preferences with patients who also want those kinds of births. And no matter what sort of nurse you have, she won't know your wishes if you don't tell her.

Creating a Hospital Postpartum Plan

If you're creating a birth plan to give the nurses and other caregivers who'll be attending your birth, you'll want to make sure to include a section on how you'd like both yourself and your baby to be treated after delivery. For example, if you're planning to breastfeed, you'll get off to a much better start if you can nurse your baby soon after birth—preferably right away. But if your care providers don't know about your wishes, they will probably follow hospital protocol instead, which may mean that your baby will be getting looked over on a warmer when you'd hoped to be nursing her.

When you're creating your postpartum birth plan, be sure to include your preferences for the following scenarios:

- If you want your baby to be with you while you're getting a tear or episiotomy repaired (if necessary), you'll want to indicate this in your postpartum plan. Also, if you'll be delivering at a teaching hospital, think about whether you'll be okay with a student performing your sutures, or if you'd rather your doctor or midwife did it.
- What do you want to happen to your placenta? If you're hoping to take your placenta home for any reason, you'll need

to let your caregivers know about this ahead of time and be sure to include it in your plan. Some hospitals won't allow you to keep the placenta.

- If you'll be breastfeeding, you'll want to make sure the nurses know not to give your baby any pacifiers or bottles of formula or sugar water, and that you'd like a visit from the hospital's lactation consultant, if there is one. Also, you may want to indicate that your baby should receive expressed breastmilk if he has to spend time in the newborn intensive care unit (NICU).

- Decide whether you'll be rooming in or rooming out. For more information on this, see Chapter 4.

- If you want your caregivers to hold off on examining your newborn until after you've had a chance to hold him and breastfeed him, make sure this is in your postpartum plan. Other routine newborn procedures, like clamping and cutting the cord, providing vitamin K injections, or putting antibiotic eye ointment on the baby can usually be delayed if you ask ahead of time.

When you create a postpartum plan, you'll need to make sure that you also communicate your wishes (or have somebody else, like a doula, your partner, or other helper, do it) to all the staff involved in your birth and postpartum experience. Remember, it's your body, your baby, and your right to ask for the treatment you want. You are a paying customer!

Creating a Support System

New moms need support and friendship, but for too many mothers, the early years of raising kids are isolated and solitary. Unfortunately, during the time when you may need the support most—when you're home with a new baby—it can be really hard to get out of the house and meet other moms. To avoid postpartum loneliness, it's a good idea to hook up with other moms during your pregnancy so you'll have a built-in support network. Here are some ways you can meet other moms:

- **Your church or religious community:** Many churches have active support groups for mothers. MOPS, or Mothers of Preschoolers, is one such support group. Check with other mothers in your church and visit Appendix B for a list of resources to try.
- **Mothering groups and classes:** Check your local community center, hospital, birth center, or continuing-education catalog for parenting classes or support groups for moms. If you're planning on breastfeeding, it's a good idea to arm yourself with encouragement and support by attending a breastfeeding class or La Leche League meeting before your baby is born. For a list of motherhood-related support groups, see Appendix B.
- **Prenatal exercise classes:** Taking a prenatal-yoga or aerobics class can do more than keep you physically healthy—it can also introduce you to a group of other expecting moms. Get to know the other women in your class, and arrange to meet up outside of class before or after your babies are born.

Of course, you don't have to start spending all your time with other expectant moms just because you're having a baby. The friends and family who are already in your life also want to be a part of your experience. The problem, however, is that the people closest to you often aren't sure how to help out, and you may not know what to ask for. This is especially true if you have friends and family who don't have their own kids. They simply may not be able to relate to what you're going through. The following are a couple of specific, fun ways you can ask others to help you prepare for a great postpartum experience:

- **Meals:** Toward the end of your pregnancy, you can throw a meal shower. Guests arrive with frozen meals that can be reheated for easy eating after your baby is born. Or invite friends over to your house and provide ingredients, a stove, and refreshments. Your friends can cook several meals for your freezer.

- **Cleaning:** You provide snacks and cleaning supplies; they provide the elbow grease. Get some friends together close to your due date to help you get your house in tiptop shape by doing the jobs you can't—like the ones that include climbing on stools or using cleaners with noxious fumes.

It's important that you communicate freely with your friends and family as your pregnancy unfolds. As long as everyone is aware of your wishes and knows how you're feeling, the people you care about most can continue being a big part of your life. All it takes is a little patience and understanding to maintain a strong support system.

Getting Help at Home and with Other Children

In the weeks after you give birth, you'll need help around the house. You'll need to rest and take it easy for a while, and you'll want to spend time just getting to know your new baby and getting used to the new demands of motherhood. This means that cooking, cleaning, and other household tasks might have to take a back seat.

If you can live with a lower level of neatness than you're used to for a while, you may be able to get by if your partner or spouse picks up some of the slack. But some women can't stand to live in a house that doesn't meet their neatness standards. If this describes you, consider hiring a cleaning service to come by a few times in the first couple of months after you give birth. This is also a great thing to add to your baby-shower registry—the gift of being able to enjoy your baby without worrying about the floors growing sticky or the bookshelves getting dusty. Or let friends and family who offer to help do the laundry, straighten up, and go shopping. You'll have an opportunity to pay them back someday.

Ľ Essential

If you don't already know any good babysitting or mother's-helper candidates, call your local middle school or Girl Scouts. Also, some community centers and YMCAs offer babysitting-readiness courses; the instructor of such a class probably has a roster of eager and trained sitters she can refer you to.

If you have older kids, you'll want to consider getting some help for their care in the early weeks after your baby is born. If you're planning on returning to work after your baby is born and your older children usually go to child care, you may not want to change things up during the postpartum weeks: Not only is it probably not a great time to disrupt an older child's schedule, but it could also make the transition harder for you.

If you will be home alone with your new baby and an older child or children, here are some ways you can make sure you get enough rest and help:

- Have Grandma and Grandpa, or an aunt, uncle, or special friend take your older child on a minivacation for a few days. This will give your older child an opportunity to feel like the center of attention again while you get a small break.
- Enroll an older child in an activity through your YMCA or community center a few hours a week. In the early weeks especially, you'll want to make sure you have a friend or family member who can do the dropping off and picking up.
- Ask a friend or family member to take your older child or children on special outings a few times a week. Running errands or going out to eat with Daddy is also a nice way to give you a break while helping an older child feel special.
- Hire a babysitter to come to the house a few hours a week. She can take older kids to the park or hold the baby for you while

you get a shower or eat a full meal. Responsible preteens and young teens can make great mother's helpers—they can play with older kids, assist with making meals, and even help out with the baby while you're close by in case she needs you.

You might also consider hiring a postpartum doula to come to your house after your baby is born. A postpartum doula is different from a baby nurse, who is usually hired to completely take over child care duties for new babies. Postpartum doulas usually don't assume responsibility of a baby's care but instead try to make caring for a baby as easy on the mother as possible. Each postpartum doula is different, but common services include light housekeeping, providing assistance with breastfeeding, caring for older children, and helping you care for your newborn. For more information on finding a postpartum doula, see Appendix B.

Stocking Up for Postpartum

You've probably thought of all the things you'll need for your new baby, but have you thought about what things might be nice to have for yourself? Just as you need to make sure all your baby's needs are met, it's equally important that you have all the tools and support necessary to keep you feeling strong, healthy, and energized during your first few weeks and months as a mom. From a good nursing pillow to a good book, there are a number of things that can make your experience more pleasant and comfortable.

Nursing Pillow

Nursing pillows can save your back and neck from strain and are a useful purchase even if you won't be breastfeeding. They make a nice perch in your lap for a sleeping or bottle-fed baby, and the doughnut-shaped type can double as a pillow to sit on if you have hemorrhoids or a painful perineum after birth. Nursing pillows are readily available at toy and baby stores or department stores like Wal-Mart and Target, and you can buy one for less than $20 and up to $50 or more. Another option is a long c-shaped body pillow that you can wrap around your body in a way that's comfortable for both you and your baby.

Rice Sock

Rice-filled pillows or socks retain heat and cold and make easy, cheap, portable, and reusable heating or cooling pads, which can be nice to use during labor or for after-delivery muscle soreness or uterine cramps. Just put rice in a clean tube sock, and tie or stitch the top shut. You can put it in the fridge, or microwave it for a couple of minutes. Adding dried herbs like peppermint or lavender will give the rice sock a nice smell. The pack is inexpensive to make and will retain heat for a long time. You may need to wrap it in a towel if it's too hot for direct skin contact at first.

Good Reading

During the early weeks postpartum, you'll be doing a lot of resting, and your baby will sleep a lot. Get some books or magazines you've been wanting to read—once your baby starts to stay awake more, you won't have nearly as much time for reading!

Check online for discounted magazine subscriptions, but be sure to place your order a couple of months in advance of your due date, since it can take six to eight weeks to receive your first issue of a magazine subscription. Some good parenting-related magazines to try include *Parenting*, *Wondertime*, and *Mothering*. Don't feel like all your reading has to be motherhood related, though—sometimes, reading up on the latest celebrity gossip or flipping through a fashion mag can help you feel a little bit connected to the "old you."

Sanitary Pads

You'll need a variety of sanitary pads for the first few weeks postpartum. Some women wear Depends or another pull-up incontinence garment for the first few days—they're more absorbent, and can be easier than messing with pads and underwear on those first days. You'll probably need overnight-absorbency pads for the first week and will then be able to switch to a lighter pad. Eventually, your bleeding will taper off so much that you may just want to wear a panty liner. Tampons aren't safe to use postpartum, so you won't need any of those.

Comfy Clothes

Most women don't jump right back into their prepregnancy clothes immediately after giving birth. Wider hips, a swollen belly, and larger breasts are just a few of the changes that may stick around for some time. Get a few pair of comfortable cotton pants with elastic or drawstring waists, and larger shirts that can accommodate your new breasts and pull up easily for nursing. Just don't spend too much money on your new garments—new motherhood can be a messy job!

Supportive Bras

You'll want to have a few supportive bras in the house that will accommodate the breast changes you'll experience when your milk comes in. Your cup size will change, probably by at least one size, in the early days of nursing, so keep that in mind while shopping. You'll want to make sure the bra is comfortable and supportive, but not tight or constricting. Push-up bras or pinching underwires can constrict milk ducts, causing clogs, breast infections, or a reduced milk supply. Breathable, 100-percent cotton bras are best, since locked-in moisture can become a breeding ground for bacteria or yeast.

Choose a bra with adjustable straps and several rows of hooks. You can also buy bra extenders—they can increase the band width of your bra by several inches and allow you to achieve a custom fit while your breasts are still fluctuating in size.

If you'll be nursing, your bra should be easy to open and close in the front with one hand. Small-breasted women sometimes prefer a soft, stretchy bra, with cups that can lift right over the breast, in place of a nursing bra. This is okay as long as the cup doesn't press on or constrict the breast.

Professional Help

To make your postpartum recovery as stress free as possible, you'll want to have the names and contact information for any professionals you may need to contact on hand and easy to access. You won't want to be digging around for phone numbers when you're trying to feed a baby and rest!

Pediatrician or Family Doctor

You'll want to figure out who your baby's doctor is going to be before he's born, and see if you can arrange for him or her to visit your baby before you leave the hospital. Otherwise, you'll get whoever is on staff at the hospital. Now is a good time to ask friends, family, or a mother's support group for recommendations. You'll want to be sure whichever doctor you choose will support your parenting philosophy and is well educated about breastfeeding—not all of them are. Also, keep in mind that you don't have to take your baby to a pediatrician if you can't find one you like. Family doctors and general practitioners are usually trained to care for all members of a family, from infancy on.

Massage Therapist

Keep handy the name and phone number of a massage therapist who's experienced in massaging pregnant and postpartum women, and call to set up an appointment for a postpartum massage soon after your baby is born. Better yet, set up the appointment before your baby is born; make it for a couple of weeks after your due date—and keep it. Massage can help relax muscles that are sore and tight after birth, or from holding and nursing your baby. It also releases endorphins that can help you relax and feel less sore, and can help you sleep better. Gift certificates for postpartum massages are a great thing to suggest to friends and family that want to give you something.

Breastfeeding Specialist

If your hospital or birth center doesn't have lactation consultants on staff, you'll want to find one before you go into labor, and you should keep her number handy in case you run into any issues. La Leche League (LLL) is another great free resource for breastfeeding problems that may arise. You might find that it's easier to reach out for this help if you go to a meeting or two before having your baby. For more information on how to find a lactation consultant or local La Leche League leader, see Appendix B.

Take Advantage of This Time

The last weeks of pregnancy can seem unbearably long as you wait for your new baby to arrive. You may not be sleeping very well due to your size, and both you and your partner will probably be anxious, wondering when you are going to go into labor. While you may feel like all you want is to finally give birth, it's important to remember that this is a special time, like any other time in your pregnancy. Don't forget to take some time for yourself and also enjoy some alone time with your partner.

Take Time for Yourself

Unless your job is physically demanding or you have a health concern, it's probably fine to keep working right up until you go into labor. But just because you can work doesn't mean you should be spending every waking minute with work. It will probably be a long time before you will have this kind of freedom again. Go shopping, to a movie, or out to dinner all by yourself. Take nice long baths, get a pedicure, or enjoy a massage.

The first few weeks after the birth will be stressful while you and your partner adjust to your new lives as parents. There will be very few moments when you'll be without your baby in your arms during that time. You need to pamper yourself now, while you still have the ability to do so. It will make a big difference later.

Alert

Any massage therapist who works on pregnant women should be aware of proper positioning, vulnerable pressure points, unusually lax muscles and joints, and other concerns that are unique to pregnant women. If you get a massage during pregnancy, be sure you use a therapist who's experienced and qualified in giving pregnancy massage.

Take Time with Your Partner

Having a baby marks the end of you and your husband or partner being just a couple and the beginning of family life. You may find it difficult to get out without the baby, or you may not want to be anywhere without him for a long time. This is why it's important to spend some quality time together with your partner, just the two of you, in these final weeks of pregnancy. Go on a "date" to a movie or out to dinner, take a drive through a scenic area on a sunny day, or do something as simple as curling up together with good books on a stormy night. The experience will give you a romantic, warm memory to recall when the going gets tough during those first few weeks of parenthood.

Last-minute Considerations

You have created your postpartum plan. You've set up a support system for yourself. You have your trusty book of phone numbers close at hand. What else do you have to do? Not much, but there are a few last-minute measures that can save you a lot of anguish when you feel that first contraction. You don't know when that contraction will come, but it's good to be as prepared as possible.

Make sure the bag you've packed to take to the hospital or birth center includes all the things you'll need to be comfortable both before and after your baby's born. Some of these items might include:

- Comfortable clothes to wear in labor if you'd like to avoid the standard-issue hospital gown
- Snacks and drinks for labor and afterward
- Phone numbers of friends, family members, and other people you may want to call to deliver the good news!
- Clothes to wear home (Be realistic. You won't be wearing your prepregnancy jeans yet!)
- Toothbrush, toothpaste, facial wash, moisturizer, contact case and solution, hairbrush, and other toiletry items
- Comfort items for labor—rice socks, massage oil or lotion, birth ball
- Nursing nightgown and bra
- Your own pillow or other special item from home

If you're having your baby at home or in a freestanding birth center, your midwife will probably have a list of items to have on hand before your baby is born. Make sure you've got whatever you'll need well in advance of your due date—labor can happen at any time in those last few weeks, and you don't want to be caught unprepared!

Now that you've planned for your birth experience, packed for the hospital, and prepared your home, you can look forward to a smooth transition and a more relaxing postpartum experience. The next chapter will tell you what to expect during the first few hours after your baby is born.

CHAPTER 2

The First Few Hours after Birth

YOU'VE DONE IT! The hard work of pregnancy and birth are over, your baby is born, and you are a mother. You've now entered the postpartum period, sometimes called the fourth trimester of pregnancy. Your body has made many changes slowly over the past nine months, but the act of giving birth has created huge changes in a much shorter time. In this chapter, you'll learn what you can expect, emotionally and physically, during the first few hours after giving birth.

The Third Stage of Labor

It may sound strange after the climactic moment of your baby's birth, but labor isn't over yet. The moment after your baby is born begins what's referred to as the third stage of labor, and ends with the delivery of the placenta. Though it's a relatively short stage, usually lasting less than half an hour, a lot happens in those few minutes.

More Contractions?

Your uterus may take a short break after pushing your baby out, but within a few minutes it'll begin contracting again. These contractions are meant to help your placenta, the soft organ that nourished your baby during your pregnancy, detach from the uterine wall and come out. This can take just a few minutes or up to a half hour or more.

What's Happening in Your Uterus

During this time your doctor or midwife may place a hand gently on your belly. This is called "guarding the uterus" and is the care provider's way of checking the progress of your placenta's separation from the uterus, and also "guarding" the area so that nobody else tries to massage or press on your uterus until the placenta is detached.

 Alert

> Nobody should massage your belly or pull on your umbilical cord until the placenta has separated from your uterine wall! If an impatient care provider tries to coax the placenta into separating before it's ready, it could cause you to bleed too much.

As your uterus shrinks and compresses the placenta, it will detach from the uterine wall. You may feel a gush of blood, some discomfort, or pressure, or you may experience a pushing urge. You and your baby can help this process along by getting him or her to nurse at your breast soon after birth. Breastfeeding releases hormones that help your uterus contract more effectively. You may not realize the placenta is ready to come out until your care provider tells you it's time to deliver it. It may seem unfair at this point, but birthing the placenta often requires some work from the mother, though sometimes it just slides out. Being upright can help, and many moms find it easiest to push the placenta out in a squatting position, though you may not be able to get upright if you have had an epidural and are still numb.

Your doctor or midwife may help you deliver the placenta with gentle traction on the umbilical cord, but nobody should ever yank or pull hard on the cord. Sometimes this part stings or burns, or it may feel uncomfortable, but the placenta is a lot smaller and squishier than your baby was—it might feel similar to a water balloon—and will come out much more easily. Your care provider will probably catch the placenta in a basin or bowl so that they can monitor the amount of blood that comes out with it.

 Essential

If you've given birth underwater, as women often do at home, in birth centers, and in some hospitals, your care provider may ask you to get out of the water to birth the placenta. Some mothers also prefer to deliver the placenta on "dry land" even after they've had a water birth.

The Placenta

After the placenta is delivered, your care provider will inspect it to make sure no pieces were left behind. You may be curious to see what the organ that's kept your baby fed and provided him with oxygen inside you looks like, so don't feel shy about asking to take a look. You may even want to take the placenta home. Many families plant their baby's placenta under a tree or use it for religious or cultural rituals. As mentioned previously, some hospitals won't allow you to take your placenta home or may require that you take it home in a formaldehyde solution. Ask ahead of time to find out your hospital's policy, and come prepared by bringing an airtight container with a lid to the hospital with you. Make sure all staff involved in your baby's birth know that you want to take the placenta home, so that nobody takes it away while you aren't looking.

Fact

Animals eat their placentas, which are rich in iron and hormones and can help prevent or stop hemorrhage and possibly mitigate postpartum depression. In many human cultures, mothers traditionally ate part of the placenta.

The Fourth Stage of Labor

The next hour is called the fourth stage of labor. If all goes well, during this time you should be getting to know your new baby. But your doctor or midwife will also want to repair any tears or your episiotomy, if you've had one, and monitor you and your baby closely to make sure you're both recovering well.

Repairing Tears and Episiotomies

During this time, your doctor or midwife will inspect your vulva, vagina, and perineum (the muscles and tissue between the vagina and anus) for tearing. If you've had an episiotomy or have a tear that requires stitching, it will be repaired now. Usually, you'll be given a shot of a local anesthetic before the stitches. You may be completely numb or you may feel some discomfort or pain depending on how extensive the tear or episiotomy and how sensitive the area.

Stitching usually takes anywhere from five to fifteen minutes. In teaching hospitals, the job of suturing a tear or episiotomy is often given to a student for practice, but this will make the stitching last longer. The first hour of your baby's life is precious time for you. If you would rather use it for getting to know him or her instead of sitting through a lengthy suturing job, you are within your rights and perfectly within reason to ask your doctor or midwife to do it instead. Or you can ask to hold your baby while you're stitched, which will make a nice distraction.

No Stitches Required

Tears are often minor enough that they don't need stitching at all. Your doctor or midwife may tell you that you have a "skid mark," which is a minor abrasion that won't need stitches, though it may sting for a while, especially when you use the bathroom.

Bleeding

Your bleeding will be carefully monitored during this first hour. In order to help your uterus contract, a care provider will massage your uterus through your belly and may watch to see how much blood comes out when your uterus contracts. This may be uncomfortable or painful if your nurse is very rough with the massage. Ask for a gentler touch if you are in pain. You can keep it "rubbed up" yourself, and keeping the baby on your chest, skin to skin, even if she isn't nursing yet, will help keep your uterus firmly contracted. This decreases your bleeding and the need for the nurses to intervene.

Essential

Rarely, a care provider may decide to check your cervix or upper vaginal area for tearing; but since it's painful and usually unnecessary, many don't do it routinely. Inspecting the cervix can be necessary if your doctor or midwife suspects there may be a tear there because of trauma to the area during birth, or if you're bleeding and your care provider can't rule out your cervix as the source of the blood.

The gushes of blood that come out during these early contractions can feel alarming, but you're usually not losing nearly as much blood as it feels like. Remember, while you were pregnant, your blood volume increased by about a factor of one half. Your body no longer needs that extra blood volume, so you can lose what might seem like a lot of blood before it becomes worrisome, and your care provider will watch your bleeding carefully, especially during the first few hours. Don't hesitate to tell your care providers anyway if you feel at all concerned.

The blood and tissue left over from pregnancy is called lochia. For the first few hours after giving birth, you can expect what seems like a lot of bright red lochia, and it may contain pieces of tissue and blood clots, which are sometimes quite large. A nurse or other caregiver may place a pad directly at your perineum to catch lochia, and you'll sit or lay on absorbent pads to soak up any extra that may spill over. For the first day after birth, sudden movement, standing up, sitting, or breastfeeding may allow lochia that's pooled in your vagina to come out all at once, so it's not unusual to feel a gush when you sit, stand, or walk. Your uterus will continue to discharge lochia for weeks after delivery. It will gradually change from red to pink, then brown, yellow, and finally white.

Essential

If you haven't already, now is a great time to get your baby on the breast. Nursing stimulates the production of oxytocin, which will help your uterus contract more efficiently and limit your postpartum bleeding. For more information about breastfeeding's benefits for Mom, see Chapter 3.

After your doctor or midwife checks for tearing, does any necessary repair work, checks the size and position of your uterus, and monitors your bleeding, a nurse or midwife will clean your perineal area and the insides of your legs with warm water. Someone may place an ice pack on your perineum, and you can change into a comfy gown or pajamas if your birthing clothes got messy. Ask for help while changing in case you get dizzy.

Your Uterus after Birth

Your uterus has stretched to many times its normal size to accommodate your growing baby, but now that your baby and the placenta are vacated the premises, your uterus must shrink back to its prepregnancy size and position. This is called involution. During the first few hours postpartum, a nurse or midwife will feel your belly regularly to check the size and position of the uterus. If it feels soft or saggy to your nurse or midwife, he or she will massage it to help it contract and firm up again.

Alert

If the uterus isn't shrinking as quickly as it should be, it could indicate that a piece of the placenta didn't come out, or that there are large blood clots in the way. For more information on retained placenta, excessive postpartum bleeding, and large blood clots, see Chapter 6.

You should feel your own belly from time to time to make sure your uterus (also called the fundus) is staying very firm. It should be about the size of a grapefruit and be in the middle of your belly, and at or lower than your bellybutton. If your uterus feels like it is up and off to the right, it means your bladder is filling and getting in the way, and you should use the bathroom. If you aren't sure how to find your uterus, ask your care provider to show you where it is and where it should be.

You'll want to get to the bathroom as soon as possible after the baby is born so that you can empty your bladder. If your bladder is full, your uterus won't be able to contract as well, and you'll bleed more and be more uncomfortable. Immediately after birth, your urethra—the opening through which you urinate—may be swollen, sore, or even feel numb, making it difficult to go. Turning on the water faucet and using a squirt bottle, often called a peri bottle, to splash warm water on the area may help. If you are still having a hard time, try putting your hand in a bowl of warm water, or try to urinate in the shower or even in a tub of water. Since it's so important that you urinate often after giving birth, your care providers may recommend a catheter if you aren't able to urinate on your own. Be aware, though, that catheters can be uncomfortable, limit your mobility, and increase your risk of developing a urinary tract infection. Ask your nurse to let you try all of the previously mentioned techniques before going the catheter route.

Essential

It's a good idea to regularly massage your own uterus by stroking your fingers firmly over your lower abdomen. After the massage, your uterus should contract and then stay firm. If it doesn't contract or goes right back to being squishy, let your care provider know.

How You May Feel Physically

After your baby is born, your body goes through enormous fast-paced changes. Your pelvic and abdominal organs start returning to their prepregnancy condition and position. Your hormones begin to adjust from supporting a pregnancy to readying your body for nursing and bonding with your baby. And you've just gone through the enormously hard work of labor and delivery, and, if you delivered by cesarean section, had major surgery. Here's how your body may feel in the hours after delivery.

Never Better

Many moms feel wonderful after giving birth. The rush of endorphins that accompany the final stages of labor act as natural painkillers, and you may feel exhilarated and blissful. Some moms have a lot of energy right after birth and may have a hard time staying "down." You may also be reveling in your newly unpregnant body and all the joys that go along with it: being able to lie on your belly again, bending forward easily, and even seeing your toes!

Tired and Sore

Labor and birth are enormously hard work. It's normal to feel tender and exhausted right after your baby is born, or for soreness to kick in later after an epidural or adrenaline rush has worn off. You may even experience soreness in places you didn't even realize were working or tensed up during labor and birth, like your shoulders or calf muscles.

Faint or Woozy

Feeling dizzy, wobbly, or faint in the early postpartum hours is not too unusual. The shift from your end-of-pregnancy blood volume and body fluid to your nonpregnant state means your cardiovascular system has a lot of work to do in adapting. When you change position from lying to sitting or from sitting to standing, take a moment to allow your body to adjust. Enlist help on those first few trips to the bathroom.

Cold and Shaky

New moms may experience shivering and shaking in the first few postpartum hours, even on the hottest days. It's thought that the body is reregulating its internal thermostat. Wrap up in blankets warmed in the dryer, or tuck heating pads around you, and snuggle your warm baby skin-to-skin to keep you both nice and toasty. Ask your care providers for blankets as often as you want them.

Afterpains

The uterine contractions that keep your uterus shrinking back to its prepregnant size may continue for several hours to several days after your baby is born, and can range from uncomfortable to quite painful. Generally, the more babies a woman has had, the more intense and long-lasting these afterpains can be, and there's often no way to know how long one will last or when the next will strike. For more information on relieving the discomfort associated with these contractions, see Chapter 3.

Effects of Medication

Most women laboring in hospitals receive some form of medication for pain management. As mentioned in Chapter 1, while anesthesia may help relieve pain during labor and birth, each option has effects that can make postpartum recovery more difficult. If you had narcotic pain relief, like Nubain or Stadol, it can make it difficult for you to fully experience the birth experience and may make it difficult for your baby to nurse well at first.

 Alert

> Women who develop pre-eclampsia, or dangerously high blood pressure, during pregnancy are sometimes given a drug called magnesium sulfate during labor and birth. If you've had "mag sulfate," as it's sometimes called, you may feel nauseous or heavily drugged, or experience swelling from water retention.

If you had an epidural during labor, you may find that your lower body stays numb for a while after birth, or your legs may be unable to support your weight for some time. You may also have a catheter inserted for some time after birth, which will limit your mobility, and possibly make it harder for you to urinate spontaneously in the early hours after it is removed. The abundant IV fluids that go along with the epidural can cause you to have swollen legs, feet, and hands for some time after giving birth.

Your Emotions

Right after the birth of your baby, it's normal to feel a range of emotions. Some women feel energized and excited, while others feel exhausted and disappointed. You may even be having conflicting emotions at the same time. Don't panic—this is normal. Do your best to focus on the joy of the moment, and remember that any discomfort or sadness you're feeling will pass in time.

Natural High

You may feel a rush of relief that the work of labor and birth is over, thrilled and elated by your baby, and triumphant over having given birth. If you're feeling "up" and energized, this might be a good time to record your birth story or have somebody jot it down as you tell it, while it's still fresh in your mind. It's amazing how quickly the details of your labor and birth can become fuzzy and out of order. Grab a blank book or your journal and start writing! If you feel more comfortable chatting about your experience, maybe a small tape recorder is the choice for you.

Afraid and Overwhelmed

Now that you've got this beautiful baby, you may be unsure how you're going to take care of her—especially if you're exhausted from labor and delivery. Try to get some rest in these early hours, and be sure to stay well fed and hydrated. Also, make sure you have plenty of support lined up for the first week or two at home with your new baby. Keeping yourself healthy and enlisting plenty of help will make the job of healing and getting to know your baby much more enjoyable, and easier.

Let Down

After the buildup of waiting for your baby, the emotionally and physically taxing work of labor, and then the climactic moment of his birth, you may find yourself feeling sad that you're no longer pregnant and have to share your baby with your husband or partner, family, friends, and the medical staff. You may also be disappointed or sad over the circumstances of your birth if you had an unexpected c-section or medical emergency arise during labor or delivery, or if your baby is having difficulties adjusting to life outside of your body and will have to spend some time in the newborn intensive care unit (NICU)—or even if everything went "perfectly." Rest and take good care of yourself during this time. Consider writing about your feelings in a journal, or discussing them with your partner, midwife, doula, or trusted caregiver.

Your Appearance

Many women look beautiful, healthy, and well rested after giving birth. After all, it's a natural event, and your body was made to do it. Still, chances are that you will notice at least a few changes to your appearance in the hours after delivery. Your eyes may be bloodshot, and sometimes you'll have broken blood vessels on your face from pushing hard. You may look tired and pale, especially if you had a long labor or are very tired, but many women look flushed and radiant. Your belly will still be quite big, and you'll look about five or six months pregnant. You may find that you walk somewhat hunched over for the first day or so. If you've had a c-section, you'll have a large scar, and often, visible stitches across your lower abdomen. All of these changes will fade with time, and you'll begin to look more and more like your prepregnant self, though some changes, like loose skin around your abdomen, or scars from stretch marks and incisions, may never completely go away.

Unfortunately, worrying that you don't look very good can make you feel even more emotional and vulnerable than you already do. To ease the situation, take some measures to make yourself feel more presentable. Have your sister or best friend brush or style your hair, or ask someone to bring you your makeup or a favorite pair of earrings. Small, familiar touches like these can make all the difference to your self-esteem.

Getting Ready for Recovery

After the first hour or two postpartum has passed, you and your husband or partner will probably be left alone for a while to settle in and get to know your new baby. Many new moms spend the bulk of this first day napping and getting nursing down. If you've given birth at home, your midwives will probably stay for a couple more hours, and if you've given birth at a freestanding birth center, you'll probably stay another four to six hours and then head home. If you've given birth in a hospital, you'll probably be there for at least another day or two.

Once you've had some time to recover from the birth, things will begin to calm down. You will probably be exhausted from the physical feat you've just performed, but you'll slowly feel your strength coming back to you. In a day or two, you may even feel ready to see visitors, such as close friends and family. Remember, though, this is your time to spend with your partner and your new baby. Take things slowly, and don't do anything before you feel ready. Chapter 3 covers what you can expect from your first week of parenthood.

The First Week after Birth

THE FIRST WEEK AFTER your baby is born is often an intensely joyful time, but it can also be confusing. You've just gone through enormous physiological changes, and now you're responsible for the care and upbringing of another human being. If you're a first-time mom, you're dealing with a major identity shift—from independent woman to responsible mother. If you're already a mom, you may be wondering if you're up to doing it all over again. Take good care of yourself and let others take care of you, too, for a peaceful and healthy first week postpartum.

How You May Be Feeling

The process of labor and birth creates endorphins, nature's pain relief, and the elation of seeing your baby for the first time may have taken your mind off any aching areas. But now that the rush has worn off a little, you may find that you're tender and sore. Even something as simple as using the bathroom can be a real chore. This section covers some helpful tips for caring for your sore spots and making your first week after birth as comfortable as possible.

Your Perineum

If you had a tear or episiotomy, you may find that your perineum is most sore the first to the third day after your baby is born. Even if you didn't tear and weren't cut, it's normal to feel some achiness in your bottom, particularly in the evening or when you're tired.

E. Essential

Between excess of breastmilk, the lochia that continues to flow for weeks after giving birth, and the extra sweat the body might still be producing to get rid of excess fluid from pregnancy, many mothers report feeling "leaky" for the first several weeks postpartum.

For a sore perineum, you'll want to alternate heat and cold therapy. Heat increases circulation, promoting healing, while cold decreases swelling and relieves pain. A nurse or other care provider may give you an ice pack for your perineum soon after delivery. When you get home, you can freeze wet maxi pads or fill rubber gloves or condoms with water and freeze them. A mix of one part alcohol to 4 parts water works well. It freezes into a slush, and adjusts to your shape better than plain frozen water. Wrap any frozen item in flannel or a wash cloth—don't put ice directly onto your skin!

Take a Bath

A warm bath can be soothing and healing for tender tissues. Your doctor or midwife may recommend holding off on a full submersion if you've had an especially deep tear or extensive episiotomy, since it can be more difficult to get in and out of the tub easily and safely. In these situations, you may be able to take a sitz bath, a shallow bath that just covers your bottom, instead. You can also use your peri bottle to squirt warm or cool water over your bottom area every time you use the bathroom.

Herbal baths are also a great way to achieve postpartum comfort. Try this recipe, hailed by midwives and herbalists for its healing and soothing properties:

2 parts comfrey leaf
1 part calendula flowers

1 part lavender flowers
1 part sea salt

Bring pot of water to boil. Turn off heat, put a large handful of herbal mix in the water, and steep for 20 to 30 minutes. Strain the herb "tea" into your bath using a fine strainer or cheesecloth (to keep the leaves out of your drain). Immerse mom and baby in a comfortably warm bath for about 20 minutes.

Question

Is it safe to bathe after I've just had a baby?
A generation ago, doctors feared that water from the bath could enter the vagina and birth canal, causing infection in the postpartum woman. But since then, research has shown that bath water does not enter the vagina, and it's generally considered safe for new mothers to soak in the tub.

You can obtain these herbs in bulk at a food co-op or natural-foods store, or by mail order. Put some of the "tea" into your peri bottle as well for a healing squirt each time you use the bathroom.

Using the Bathroom
When you use the bathroom, urine may come into contact with tears, abrasions, or stitches in your perineum. It may really sting for a few days. Concentrated urine stings more than regular-strength urine when it comes into contact with traumatized tissue, so be sure to drink enough fluids. Keep using your peri bottle to squirt warm water or the herbal recipe on your vaginal area each time you use the bathroom. Pat yourself dry when you're done using the toilet, always moving the toilet tissue from front to back.

You will probably notice that you have to pee a lot in the first days after giving birth. Your body is ridding itself of excess fluids it no longer needs. Be sure to keep your bladder empty, as a full bladder will make afterpains (uterine contractions) worse, make it more difficult for your uterus to contract, and can lead to a bladder infection. If you are still finding it difficult, you can try urinating in the shower or even while in the bath. Your urine is sterile when it comes out, so you don't have to worry about your urine "infecting" your healing body. You may find it hard to tell when your bladder is full in the first days, so try to urinate every hour or so while you are awake, whether you feel like it or not, until the sensation is all back. If you aren't able to urinate, feel pain or burning during or after urination (except for the stinging you may feel when your urine touches abrasions, tears, or your episiotomy site), or if you feel like you have to urinate even when your bladder is empty, call your care provider.

 Alert

In the first few days after giving birth, you may find that you leak urine when you sneeze or cough. This condition is called stress incontinence, and should improve after your bladder and other internal organs have gotten back into their prepregnancy condition. Sometimes, though, incontinence lasts past the postpartum period.

Sometime in the first few days after giving birth, you will probably need to have a bowel movement. This can be scary the first time. A lot of mothers would rather not push anything out of their bodies so soon after birth, and you may also fear that you will reopen a wound. But you'll find that it's not nearly as bad as you're afraid it will be. You can try applying a little pressure to your perineum with a piece of gauze, toilet paper, or Tucks pad. This might make it a little easier to empty your bowels and will also help you feel as though you're protecting any healing tears or stitches, though you really don't have to worry that having a bowel movement will reopen stitches. Give yourself some time, don't strain, and try some deep breathing exercises if you are having a hard time relaxing on the toilet. Eating a diet high in fiber and making sure you drink enough fluids can help your stools stay soft and help you pass them easily. If you haven't had a bowel movement within a few days of having your baby, call your health-care provider.

Hemorrhoids

Hemorrhoids are varicose veins, or swollen blood vessels, in the rectal area. Pregnant women are prone to varicosities of all sorts due to sluggish circulation, and hemorrhoids are often caused or exacerbated by the weight of the baby on the pelvic region during the last weeks of pregnancy. They can also be caused or worsened by the pressure of your baby's head as he is pushed out past the perineum.

Hemorrhoids can itch, burn, or hurt, and they may bleed, particularly during a bowel movement. They may be just under the skin or protrude through the anus and get as large as the size of a grape.

Be sure to give your rectal area a squirt with the peri bottle each time you use the bathroom, then pat—don't rub or wipe—the area dry, always moving from front to back. Medicated, premoistened wipes made for hemorrhoids might be more comfortable for wiping after using the bathroom. Use Tucks pads or cotton balls dipped in witch hazel to help hemorrhoids shrink, and to soothe the area. Be sure to check with your care provider before using any medicated suppositories or other hemorrhoid creams.

Ⅼ, Essential

Many women rave about Dermoplast, an over-the-counter analgesic spray that can help numb tissue and soothe hemorrhoids. Some experts say you shouldn't spray Dermoplast directly on the site of a tear or episiotomy, so ask your doctor or midwife before you use it for that purpose.

If you have hemorrhoids, it might make you especially reluctant to have a bowel movement. If you're really afraid, using hemorrhoid cream that contains topical anesthetic can soothe and lubricate the area and make it more comfortable to move your bowels. If you have hemorrhoids, it is especially important that you don't get constipated. Be vigilant with your diet, avoiding constipating foods like processed cereals and bread. If a hemorrhoid is bleeding all the time, or getting bigger, or the pain is intolerable, call your doctor or midwife.

Bleeding

As mentioned previously, your bleeding will continue during this first week. Sometimes lochia turns from red to pink to brown and lightens, only to become red and heavier again. This usually means you are doing too much too soon.

Organ Movement

During pregnancy, your internal organs gradually shift around to make room for your growing baby. Then, when your baby is suddenly gone from your uterus, your organs have to make their way back to their prepregnancy position. This can make you feel like your organs are just hanging in space. This feeling will pass over the next week or so, as your abdominal muscles regain some of their tone and your organs shift back into place. A support garment made especially for supporting your pelvis and abdomen during the postpartum weeks may help.

Dealing with Afterpains

If this is not your first baby, you may experience uterine cramping or afterpains. These pains may continue through much of the first week postpartum. Mothers sometimes complain that afterpains are actually worse than labor contractions, and they may seem to go on for a much longer time with no predictable pattern. It seems especially unfair that they're so painful considering that you've already done all the work of labor and birth. Don't worry; there are several things you can do to lessen the discomfort of these contractions:

- **Prevention:** Be sure to urinate frequently. A full bladder can make afterpains happen more frequently and be much more painful.
- **Pressure:** Lying on your belly or wrapping your abdomen with an Ace bandage, sling, or support garment made specifically for postpartum abdominal and pelvic support can help keep everything in place and make afterpains less intense.
- **Heat:** Placing a heating pad, a warm rice sock, a hot water bottle, or your nice warm baby on your belly is a great way to relieve uterine cramps. Try lying on your stomach, with the heating pad underneath your belly—the combination of heat and pressure can make even the most severe afterpains bearable.
- **Relaxation exercises:** If you learned breathing techniques for labor or practiced birth hypnosis, you can use those methods to help you through postpartum uterine contractions. If you didn't learn any special breathing techniques, try taking slow, deep breaths when you feel an afterpain coming, and try to relax your muscles. If that doesn't work, you can try taking a deep breath in, then panting on your exhale. Ask your husband or partner to massage your shoulders during afterpains, since massage can release endorphins into your blood stream and help reduce your perception of pain.

If none of these measures is working for you, you still have one more option: pain medication. Talk to your doctor or midwife about taking pain medication to take the edge off the contractions. Also, read the next section, which covers medical pain relief in greater detail.

Medical Pain Relief

If you've had your baby in a hospital, there will likely be an array of pain-relief options available for your postpartum stay, and you will probably have the option of taking a supply home with you. Each drug has its own positives and negatives, though, so be sure you understand what you're taking and what effects it might have.

Over-the-counter Painkillers and Anti-inflammatory Drugs

For all-over soreness and uterine cramping, taking ibuprofen and acetaminophen (most commonly called Advil or Motrin, and Tylenol) around the clock are popular choices. Both of these drugs are generally considered safe to take while nursing. Often, one medication will begin to wear off before you can take another dose of that same medication. If this happens, you may take ibuprofen and acetaminophen together so that one is kicking in just as the other is wearing off, and you can alternate the two so that as one is wearing off, the other is just kicking in.

Essential

In the first few days after having a baby, it's easy to forget when you had your last dose of medication, especially if you're alternating painkillers. Try creating a simple chart and keeping it by your bed or sofa, then checking off each medication as you take it to keep you from accidentally skipping or doubling up on a dose.

If you're taking acetaminophen, it's important that you not exceed the dosage recommended on the label, because of the danger of liver damage. But most women can safely take ibuprofen at a dosage of 800 mg every four to six hours, as long as they don't exceed 2,400 mg in a twenty-four-hour period. You shouldn't need it for more than two or three days—if you do, talk to your midwife or doctor about dosage. If you choose to take these medications, you'll want to make sure to keep up the dosage around the clock to keep pain at bay. If you wait until the pain is most intense, the medication may not have as much effect.

Something Stronger

If you're very sore, your doctor, midwife, or a nurse may offer you Tylenol 3, which contains codeine. This is usually considered safe, but as with any narcotic, be careful—some people react more strongly to pain-relieving medications than others. Some health-care providers routinely give new mothers strong medications like Vicodin to manage soreness. If you're recovering from a c-section, are in a lot of pain, and can't enjoy your new baby or get any sleep, you may consider these options. However, be aware that these medications may have negative effects. Some of these medications are constipating, which can make after-birth cramping and hemorrhoids worse. You may also find that you're very drowsy and unable to hold your baby, and you may also fall into a deep sleep and have a hard time waking up to feed or care for her. Ask your care provider about side effects before you take any medications, and if drowsiness is a side effect, be sure you have another person in the room to help you care for your baby.

Caring for Stitches

If you've had stitches or a tear, your bottom will be sore, itchy, or both for a few days to a few weeks after delivery. Increasing circulation to the area can help promote healing, so keep taking warm baths or sitz baths a few times a day. Keeping your legs together as much as you can helps small tears heal quicker and keeps stitches from getting pulled. Also, try to expose your perineum to the air for at least a while every day. This will aid in healing. Try putting 1 cup of salt into your bathwater if not using herbs. This will help the area to heal, and also will help make stitches feel less itchy or pulling.

Try to return to doing Kegel exercises, which can increase circulation to the perineal area, aid with healing, and strengthen your pelvic floor, as quickly as you can after giving birth. To perform Kegel exercises, gently tighten your perineal muscles as if you were trying to stop urinating. Slowly pull the muscles up as tightly as you can, hold for a few seconds, and slowly release. Start with five at a time—it's more important to do them frequently than to do large numbers of repetitions all at once. At first, you may have a hard time feeling your pelvic-floor muscles enough to tighten them, and you may feel sore. Applying gentle pressure to the area might help you locate the muscles you're trying to tighten.

 Alert

To prevent infection in your healing perineum, wash your hands before and after you use the bathroom. Always wipe front to back to avoid moving bacteria from your rectum into your healing tissues, and change your sanitary pad each time you use the bathroom, since pads can harbor bacteria.

Sitting on a doughnut pillow or on two pillows, with one buttock on each and a space between to allow for your perineum, may be more comfortable while your stitches heal. Or you can try sitting straight down on your bottom to avoid pulling. Experiment and find out which positions feel best to you.

If your perineum feels worse from day to day instead of better, if the swelling gets worse, if it looks like a repaired episiotomy or tear is separating, if you notice a foul smell or pus coming out of stitches, or if the area around stitches becomes red or looks bruised, call your midwife or doctor.

Handling Visitors

Most new moms want to show off their babies, and friends and family may be eager to stop by, see your new little one, and offer their congratulations. But it's easy to become overexerted by a constant stream of visitors in these early days. Guests during this time should be eager to help you, not the other way around. Don't feel like you have to play hostess to visitors. Ask friends and family to help you out by bringing a meal with them when they visit, washing a sinkful of dishes, or putting a load of laundry in the washing machine, instead of letting them coo over the baby while you do chores. Limit the length of visits—your baby might become overstimulated by too much passing around, and you need to rest as much as you can. Also, be sure that your older children don't get overlooked during these visits. Though your loved ones may be eager to see the new baby, remind them to pay some attention to older children, too.

 Fact

Feeling weepy, anxious, moody, or "fuzzy" during the first weeks after giving birth is called the baby blues. Hormonal fluctuations, stress, and lack of sleep can all add to the baby blues, which will eventually go away without treatment. You may also feel like telling your birth story over and over to anyone who will listen, or it's possible that you won't be ready to talk about your birth or look at birth pictures yet. It's normal to feel either way.

You may not feel comfortable asking certain guests to run errands for you or letting them know when you need to rest, especially if it's someone you have a strained or tense relationship with. It may be best not to have that person in your home at all in these first weeks. But if you can't get around it, try setting up an endpoint to the visit ahead of time. Let the guest know—or have your husband or partner let him or her know—that you have another appointment or commitment in an hour, so the visit will have to be brief. And if you're feeling pressured, you can always make your midwife or doctor be the "bad guy" who requires you to limit your visitors and visits.

Why Breastfeed?

Your doctor or midwife has probably already told you about the many benefits of breastfeeding where your baby is concerned, but you may not know that nursing also offers mothers a host of benefits. When you nurse your baby immediately after birth, the nuzzling and sucking helps release oxytocin, which creates contractions that can prevent postpartum hemorrhage and also help the uterus return to its prepregnancy state quicker.

Breastfeeding helps delay the return of your period and can act as a natural form of child spacing as long as a baby is nursing exclusively, frequently, and through the night (without getting formula, food, or a pacifier). Most women will be infertile with this kind of nursing, especially in the early days, though like any method, breastfeeding is not 100 percent effective. For more information about the lactational amenorrhea method (LAM) of contraception, see Chapter 11. Delaying your period will also help your body retain its iron stores and reduce the risk of iron-deficiency anemia. Studies suggest that the calories burned during nursing—between 200 and 500 per day—can help nursing mothers lose pregnancy weight more quickly.

 Fact

Breastfeeding moms enjoy many long-term health benefits. Studies have shown that breastfeeding can lead to a lower risk of heart disease, osteoporosis, and reproductive cancers like ovarian, cervical, and uterine cancers. Breastfeeding also cuts a woman's risk of breast cancer drastically. Breastfeeding for two years has been shown to reduce the risk of breast cancer by 50 percent.

Breastfeeding may also make you feel good—the hormones that help your body produce milk, oxytocin and prolactin, can induce a state of calmness and help you relax. They're also associated with the strong sense of love mothers often feel for their newborn babies and can both help prevent the baby blues and promote bonding with your baby. And, of course, breastfeeding is free, travels easily, and many new moms find it more convenient than the bottle washing, mixing, and heating that go along with formula feeding.

Breastfeeding frequently over the first few days will help your milk come in more quickly, and it will help your body learn how much milk to make to satisfy your baby. When you nurse frequently—when your baby wants to, rather than on a rigid schedule—it will help your mature milk come in on time, usually between the second and fifth day after your baby is born.

Beginning Breastfeeding

The first few nursing sessions can be tricky. You may be new at this, and certainly your baby is. Even a woman who has breastfed before may be surprised by a very different baby than her others. Nature is on your side here, so be patient with yourself and your baby. Take your time. Offer your breast every time the baby signals interest by moving his mouth, smacking his lips, nuzzling his face against you, or chewing his fist. Try not to wait until the baby is really hungry. If you or your baby become frantic, stop, cuddle, and calm down. Try taking off your top and bra so you have less to fuss with. If you're having trouble getting your baby to latch on, don't panic. It doesn't always go smoothly at first, but with persistence and support, breast-feeding can almost always work.

Perfecting the Latch

The foundation of a successful breastfeeding experience is a comfortable nursing position and a good latch. If this is your first child, this whole breastfeeding thing is going to seem very new to you. Luckily, it's a natural part of caring for your baby, and most people find it's smooth sailing after a few initial bumps. Follow these steps for success:

1. **Get comfortable.** You should be sitting or lying in a relaxed position, with your arms, back, and neck well supported.

2. **Make sure you're tummy to tummy with your baby.** He should be level with your breast—use pillows to boost him if necessary—and his face and body should both be turned toward you. It's very difficult for a baby to suck and swallow if his face is turned toward you but his body is turned away. Make sure his ear, shoulder, and hip are aligned.

3. **Hold your breast in one hand, and your baby's head with the other.** Try holding your breast with a "C"-hold: with the weight of your breast in your hand, wrap your thumb around the top of your breast, just behind the areola. This position will help you support and control your breast and make it easier to get enough areola into your baby's mouth.

4. **Wait until your baby's mouth is open wide.** Tickling his cheek or bottom lip will stimulate his rooting reflex and may encourage him to open his mouth.

5. **If your baby likes to try to get his hands in his mouth, it can make getting a good latch difficult.** Try swaddling your baby so that his arms are held down at his sides, or enlist help.

6. **Pull your baby onto your breast with your nipple pointed at the roof of his mouth.** Make sure you bring the baby to you, rather than hunching or leaning over to put your breast in his mouth.

If at any time you think your baby isn't latched on correctly, break the latch and try again. To break the suction, insert your finger into the corner of his mouth and pull away from your breast. If you try to pull your nipple out of your baby's mouth without breaking the suction first, it can really hurt.

Try these methods:

- **Look at your baby's lips.** They should both be visible. If either lip is tucked in along with your nipple, break the latch and start again.

- **Pull back your baby's lip to check whether his tongue is positioned properly.** It should cover his lower gum line. If your baby's tongue is making a clicking sound while he nurses, or you can't see his tongue at all, he may be sucking it along with your nipple. Break the latch and start again.
- **If you think your baby is sucking on his tongue,** or if it doesn't look like he has a good latch with at least an inch of areola in his mouth, **break the latch and start again**.

Breastfeeding at Home

Breastfeeding when you're back in your own house can feel very different from the hospital, where you may have been surrounded by helpers or had an uncomfortable sense of performance anxiety. If you had a stressful experience in the hospital because of unsupportive nurses or that feeling of being in a fishbowl, you can relax: you're on your own turf now, and you and your baby can work this out even if you got off to a rough start. If you're feeling a little anxious about going this alone without the guidance of trained medical staff, remember that women have been nursing babies since the beginning of time.

L. Essential

If you won't be breastfeeding, you'll want to wear a snug bra or bind your breasts with stretchy bandages for the first few days postpartum. And even if you're not breastfeeding, you can still make each feeding a time for bonding. Hold your baby close to your body while you feed her, and try unbuttoning or removing your shirt during some feedings so you get the skin-to-skin contact you and she will both crave.

Your Nursing Nook

First, make sure you set yourself up for relaxing and successful nursing sessions at home. Have you eaten and used the bathroom recently? You may be here a while. Be sure your hands are clean—you'll probably have to get them in or near your baby's mouth again and again. Find a place in your home that will become your nursing nook: a comfortable chair, your bed, or a corner of the sofa. Stock the area with your breastfeeding supplies: a pillow, rolled-up blanket, or other support for your arms, elbows, and baby; water (breastfeeding will make you very thirsty!); magazines or a book; the phone; a stool, stack of books, or something else to rest your feet on; a cloth diaper or towel to catch spraying or leaking milk or spit-up; and anything else you might need. The first few weeks postpartum may begin to feel like one long nursing session—use it as a time to relax, nibble a nutritious snack, sip water or herbal tea, and read a good book.

When Your Milk Comes In

You'll notice that your baby follows a pattern when she nurses. She'll suck faster and more aggressively at first to stimulate the milk-ejection reflex. When your milk comes in, usually sometime between day two and five postpartum, your milk will "let down" or begin flowing after a few minutes of this rapid sucking. When the milk comes out, your baby will switch to a slower sucking pattern, punctuated by swallows, which you can usually hear. Some women don't feel their milk letting down at all, while others feel a tingling or pins-and-needles sensation. Either is normal.

L. Essential

If your baby begins sputtering or coughing after your milk lets down, you may have a very abundant supply or a fast milk-ejection reflex. Remove your baby from the breast until she stops coughing and swallows, and then latch on again. As she matures, your baby will be better equipped to handle a fast flow of milk.

Two Kinds of Milk

The milk your baby is swallowing at first is your foremilk, which is usually thin and looks bluish or watery. It can come out very quickly, especially at first, and your baby may leak quite a bit of it while she's getting the hang of swallowing. After a few minutes, your breast will begin to produce hindmilk, a thick, creamy milk that's higher in fat and nutrients and helps your baby feel full longer. If you switch breasts too soon, your baby may not get enough of the hindmilk, which can lead to gassiness and an overabundant milk supply. Be sure your baby "finishes" the first breast by nursing until she's done. The "rule" of nursing for only ten minutes on one side, then switching, is outdated. New research shows that your baby needs to get her fill of the fatty, nutrient-rich hindmilk that comes later in the feeding. Watch your baby, not the clock. Let her finish one side, burp her, and then switch to the other breast. If she's fallen asleep or isn't interested, be sure to start with the "unused" breast next time. For help with troubleshooting common breastfeeding problems and more information about caring for your breasts over the coming weeks and months, see Chapter 8.

CHAPTER 4

Your Hospital Stay

THE DAYS YOU SPEND in the hospital after your baby is born should be a restful, happy time for you and a chance to settle in to your role of mom with lots of support and help. But your hospital stay will also be full of paperwork, procedures, and protocol, all of which can be overwhelming. This chapter will help you sort through everything you need to know to get the most out of your hospital stay.

What to Expect from Hospital Staff

Once upon a time, new mothers stayed in the hospital for several days to a week after their babies were born. Because of pressure from insurance companies and efforts to keep costs down, the post-partum stay is now usually one or two days long, at most, when the birth is normal and the mother and baby are both doing fine. For a mom with lots of knowledge and support, recovering at home is often preferable. But for many mothers, the hospital stay will be the only opportunity to be cared for and to have all questions and concerns addressed until the follow-up visit in four to six weeks. Since there are many questions and issues that can come up during the early postpartum weeks, it's very important to make sure you have ample support at home and really understand how to care for yourself before you leave the hospital.

Procedures and Tests

During your hospital stay, nurses will routinely take your blood pressure and pulse, check your bleeding, and ask how you're feeling. They will continue to feel your uterus to make sure it's staying firm, check to make sure you are using the bathroom regularly, and may offer you assistance with breastfeeding.

If your blood's RH factor is negative and your baby's father's is positive, you've probably already talked with your doctor or midwife about receiving Rh-immune globulin (RhoGAM) after your baby is born. A blood test from you and a sample of your baby's blood, taken from the umbilical cord, will tell your doctor or midwife whether you'll need a postpartum shot of RhoGAM. If you do, it will be administered during your hospital stay.

Security

Due to heightened security measures, many mother and baby units now have elaborate systems in place to keep your baby from leaving the hospital without you. At the very least, you will probably be given identification bracelets with numeric codes matching you to your baby. Some hospitals will attach an alarm that uses wireless technology to keep track of where your baby is at all times, and it may set off an alarm and automatically lock security doors if anyone tries to remove the alarm or take the baby out of the mother-baby unit.

 Alert

Your hospital may have a system in place that will help you identify staff. Don't ever hand your baby to anyone if you aren't 100 percent sure he or she is hospital staff. If you aren't sure, call for your nurse.

The hospital may also take a photo of your newborn for security purposes. Most hospitals also have rules about how babies may be transported in the hallways, and who may carry them. If you don't understand your hospital's security procedures, be sure to ask a nurse to explain them. Many parents have accidentally set off security alarms by walking too close to an open door with their baby.

Eating Healthfully in the Hospital

It's important to eat a healthy, nutritious diet containing plenty of fiber when you've just had a baby. Hospital fare can be constipating, and the meals are not always substantial enough to support a nursing mother's need for 200 to 500 extra calories per day. If you get a choice of menu from the hospital cafeteria, choose the foods that seem freshest and contain whole grains, fruits, or vegetables. Try to include foods containing iron, like leafy green vegetables or red meat, to restore your iron levels, which may be low due to blood naturally lost after birth.

Essential

Some hospitals have dieticians that routinely speak to patients about eating healthfully, or may work with you to pick the best choices for you from the hospital menu. This may be especially helpful if you have a condition like high blood pressure or diabetes.

Often, mother and baby units will stock special snacks including yogurt, fruit, and cheese for new moms in a refrigerator near the nurse's station. Don't hesitate to ask your nurse for more food if you're still hungry after eating a meal, or to send your spouse or partner out for more food if there isn't anything available in the hospital, or they don't offer what you really want. Also, don't forget to drink plenty of water! Call for a nurse to bring you snacks or something to drink if you need it. This is your time to rest and be cared for.

Rooming In Versus Rooming Out

If your hospital has a newborn nursery and your baby is healthy and full term, you may be given the option of rooming out (keeping your baby in the nursery) instead of rooming in (keeping your baby in your hospital room with you all or most of the time). A generation ago, rooming out was much more common, but now it's much rarer to find a hospital that doesn't allow, or sometimes even encourage, babies to room with their mothers during the hospital stay. There are several reasons not to use the rooming-out option if it's offered to you.

Breastfeeding Success

Rooming out can make breastfeeding on demand difficult, since you can't watch the baby for signs of hunger like smacking lips and rooting for a nipple. And since nursing frequently in the first few days is key to breastfeeding success and preventing engorgement, not being near your baby most of the first few days can lead to engorged, sore breasts and nipple pain down the road, which can make nursing much more difficult. Also, if your baby is away from you, there's a much greater chance she'll be given a bottle in the nursery, and this can lead to difficulty with breastfeeding.

 Alert

If you choose to let your baby go to the newborn nursery during your hospital stay and you're breastfeeding, make sure nurses put a sign in your baby's bassinet that he's not to be given any sugar water, formula, bottles, or pacifiers; as mentioned previously, all of these can make nursing more difficult.

Gaining Confidence and Mothering Skills

It is easier to establish yourself, emotionally and practically, as your new baby's mother if you have a chance to get to know her and feel in control of her care. Taking over most of your baby's care while in the hospital lets you learn how to comfort, feed, and care for her while there's still a lot of help nearby. If you keep your baby with you all or most of the time, you'll start to notice her eating, sleeping, diapering, and waking patterns, and begin to distinguish between her different cries, figuring out which ones mean she's hungry, which ones mean she's wet, and so on.

If you aren't sure how to feed, hold, or change your baby, this is a perfect opportunity to learn. Ask a nurse for help if you need to the first couple of times, but assume responsibility for figuring out when your baby needs to be fed or changed, and gradually take over the tasks yourself. That way, you'll establish confidence and authority in yourself as your baby's mother *before* you leave the hospital.

A Boon for Bonding

Babies are biologically programmed to begin bonding at birth, and when you keep your baby close by you, you can facilitate a connection that will make the early months of her life more enjoyable for both of you. Also, if your baby is away from you in a newborn nursery or at the nurse's station, you may feel anxious about the separation or worry about whether your baby is doing okay.

But if your baby can't be with you right now because she needs to spend some time in the NICU, don't worry that you can never bond with her. As long as you're recovering well, you should be able to make frequent visits to the NICU to see and possibly hold and feed your baby. Remember, bonding isn't something that happens all at once—it's a process that will unfold as you and your baby come to know each other.

Getting Enough Sleep

Don't worry too much that you won't be able to get any rest if you keep your baby with you in your hospital room. Newborn babies sleep a lot, and you will likely have plenty of opportunities for rest if you nap when your baby naps. If you are exhausted and afraid you won't wake up if your baby cries, ask your husband or partner or a close family member or friend to hold her while you take a nap. If you don't have anyone in the hospital with you who can hold the baby, you can have a nurse take her just after she's eaten. That way, you can get a nap in with the knowledge that your baby is, for now, full and content. If you're breastfeeding, make sure the nurse knows to bring the baby back if she starts showing any signs of hunger.

Personal and Professional Visitors

During your hospital stay, you can expect a variety of guests, from family and friends eager to see your baby and wish you well to the hospital staff members who'll pay you a visit or two before you're discharged. Depending on where you give birth, there may be several different guidelines or rules in place regarding visitors. Always check with your hospital or birth center well in advance of your due date to make sure you understand their visitor policies.

Family and Friends

Most hospitals will allow you and your baby to have visitors during specific hours. There may be rules about how many visitors you can have at one time, or about whether children are allowed to visit you. If you have other children, they will probably want to come see you in the hospital and meet their new baby brother or sister, so find out what your hospital's policy is on children visitors ahead of time. Be sure not to tire yourself by having too many people visiting during these early days. On the other hand, some women find that having visitors in the hospital rather than at home can be more relaxing, since they are on neutral territory and don't feel as though they have to play hostess or clean up before the company arrives. Also, having some of your visitors come to the hospital instead of your house makes it easy to keep the visitors from staying on and on—you can always use visiting hours or an upcoming examination from a nurse as an excuse for cutting a visit short.

Professional Visitors

In addition to your friends and family, you can expect visits from a few professionals during your hospital stay. If you qualify for any social services or state aid, such as food stamps, Medicaid, or WIC, you may get a visit from a social worker, who may ask you about your home environment, other children, your partner, and other personal questions. The social worker may also ask whether you want home services or help with transportation to medical appointments for you and your baby.

Ļ. Essential

Your hospital may also employ clergy, like a pastor, priest, or rabbi, that may make a visit routinely or by your request. If you've indicated a specific religion on your hospital registration papers, you may be offered a visit by a leader from your religious organization. Some clergy will perform blessings for new babies before they go home from the hospital.

At some point, your midwife or doctor will check on you and see how your healing is progressing. If your doctor or midwife works in a practice with others, the person who visits you postpartum may not be the same person who attended your birth. Be sure to discuss any concerns you have about your healing with your care provider, since you may not see him or her again until your follow-up visit in four to six weeks.

As mentioned previously, if you chose your baby's pediatrician or family doctor before you gave birth, he or she may examine your baby before you check out of the hospital. Otherwise, a hospital pediatrician will usually visit your baby—and have a chat with you—before you are discharged.

Help with Breastfeeding

Many hospitals employ a lactation consultant, or breastfeeding specialist, to help you get off to a good start nursing your baby. Sometimes, hospital breastfeeding specialists routinely visit new moms, but sometimes they make visits by request only. If you had a midwife for your birth, she should be knowledgeable about breastfeeding and willing to help. If you are having a hard time with breastfeeding and feel like you need some special help—or just want some pointers for nursing successfully once you're home—don't hesitate to ask whether your hospital has a lactation expert you can speak with. If they don't have a lactation expert available, you may be able to get a La Leche League volunteer to visit you in the hospital. For more information on breastfeeding, lactation consultants, and La Leche League, see Appendix B.

Your Own Customer-service Specialist

Your hospital may also have a patient liaison, a person whose job is to act as a buffer between patients and staff and make sure your needs and wishes are met during your stay. If you have trouble with a specific member of the hospital staff or are unhappy with any aspect of your care, it may be easier to talk to a third party than to directly confront the medical staff.

Keep in mind that you can refuse any visitor you don't want to see, or ask them to come back at another time. One of your rights as a patient is to choose your caregivers, which means that you can ask for a new nurse or doctor if you aren't comfortable with one who's assigned to you. In a teaching hospital, resident doctors do the bulk of the care. If you are willing to help train the doctors and nurses of the future, please do—but be aware that you have the right to ask for the care you want. Take a "consumer" approach to your health care—remember, it's a service you are paying for, even if your insurance company is picking up the tab. You have a right to feel well cared for and respected by the hospital staff.

Paperwork

During your hospital stay, you'll have plenty of paperwork to fill out, including informed consent forms for certain medical procedures or tests you or your baby may undergo, a release form that allows the hospital to send details like your baby's day and time of birth to the newspaper for a birth announcement, and a worksheet that will be used to create your baby's official birth certificate. Keep in mind that if you are married but do not share your husband's last name, you may be required to show a marriage certificate before the hospital will add him to the birth certificate. Look over all paperwork carefully before you sign it. An incorrect birth certificate can be a hassle to fix later.

 Alert

In some hospitals, the staff will start putting paperwork under your nose very soon after your baby is born to get it done and out of the way. This is bad timing for most moms, who just want to enjoy their babies! Let nurses know that you'd like to fill out your paperwork later—it can wait.

In many states you can opt to sign your baby up for a social security number when you sign the birth-certificate worksheet. The hospital won't be able to issue you a copy of your baby's social security card or an official birth certificate. Ask your hospital for the names of the local offices where you can request a copy of these documents. They should be able to supply you with contact information. In many states, you can now request copies of your baby's birth certificate online, but it will take some time to be processed.

If You Are Unmarried

If you are not married to your baby's father, he may be required to sign an acknowledgment or affidavit that he is the baby's father (sometimes called paternity papers) before he can be included on your baby's birth certificate, or sometimes before you can legally give your baby his last name. Your hospital should have information available about paternity laws in your state, but it's a good idea to find out beforehand what you'll need to do to complete your baby's birth certificate.

You can, however, legally file your baby's birth certificate without naming a father. If you aren't sure who the father of your baby is, if he's not involved in your life, if he is abusive or dangerous, or if you are in a same-sex couple and became pregnant through artificial insemination, you may not be willing or able to name a father on your baby's birth certificate.

Essential

If you are raising your baby with a same-sex partner, you will probably leave the "father's information" section of the birth certificate blank. Depending on your state's laws, your partner may be able to adopt your baby later and have her name added to the birth certificate.

If you are pressured to give information about your baby's father to a social worker or hospital staff, know your rights. In many states, it is not legal to force women to name the father of their baby to receive social services like Medicaid. Be aware that naming a father to a social worker will often start paternity proceedings, which may force an unwilling father to pay child support or compensate the state for money spent on health care during your pregnancy or for medical coverage, cash assistance, or child-care subsidies for your baby. While practical and financial support for you and your child are important, you may have many reasons for not wanting to draw an unwilling parent into your and your baby's lives during this vulnerable time. Protect yourself and your baby, and do not be bullied into signing anything if you don't feel like it's the right thing to do.

The Name Game

Some moms aren't sure what they want to name their baby right away, and may experience some pressure in the hospital to hurry up and pick a name so the birth certificate can get filed. Legally, you are not required to choose a name for your baby before you leave the hospital, but be aware that your hospital is required by law to submit a birth certificate for your baby, even if it means they have to leave the first and middle names blank.

Insurance and Other Benefits

Don't forget to check with your insurance provider to find out what kind of documentation you'll need, if any, from the hospital to add your baby to your policy. Also be sure you understand what services are covered under your insurance policy. Your insurance may not cover some procedures, like infant circumcision, and it may not pay for a private room. If you're using short-term disability leave, paid maternity leave, or the Family Medical Leave Act, it's a good idea to call your employer now to make sure all your paperwork is in order. Better yet, have your spouse or partner make the call for you.

When You'll Be Released

Sometime between a day and two days after your baby is born, you'll probably be released from the hospital. You may stay longer if your baby was born via c-section or if your doctor or midwife decides you need more time to recover, which may be the case if you had a difficult or complicated birth. If you don't feel well enough to leave the hospital, be sure to communicate this to the hospital staff.

When it's time for you to leave the hospital, you may be offered a bag of formula samples. If you'll be breastfeeding, there's no need for you to accept these, since formula and bottles in the early weeks of nursing can undermine your milk supply and make nursing more difficult. Of course, you can keep the goodies—like the diaper bag, breastmilk-collection containers, and freezer packs—and leave the formula behind.

L. Essential

A baby's hospital bassinet is often stuffed full of goodies like bulb syringes (the hospital type works much better than the kind you can buy at the drugstore), diapers, and samples of baby toiletries. Ask if you can take some of these items home—often, the nurses will tell you to take it all.

When you're being discharged from the hospital, they'll disengage any security systems your baby might be attached to, and a nurse will probably walk with you to the exit. You may have to ride to the exit in a wheelchair if that is your hospital's policy. Most hospitals will not allow you to leave with your baby if you do not have an infant car safety seat with you. If you don't have and can't afford a car seat, the hospital may be able to provide you with one for free, but you'll need to look into this option ahead of time to make sure everything is ready for you before you check out. A nurse may check to make sure your car seat is installed properly before you leave. Make sure you know who to call if you have any questions or concerns once you get home.

If Your Baby Has to Stay

If your baby isn't going to be released from the hospital on the same day as you, the reason is probably that your baby is premature or sick. A range of feelings can be normal if your baby is sick or premature—sadness, fear, anxiety, guilt, and even disconnection. You'll probably be anxious about your baby's health and, if you had a difficult birth, may be grieving over that experience as well.

If your baby has to stay in the hospital for a while, ask how you can stay close to your baby while she's there. Many NICUs have a place for moms and dads to sit with the baby, and your hospital may offer a "hospitality" room with a bed for you, and maybe your spouse or partner, to sleep in at night.

You Are the Mother

Moms with sick or premature babies often find themselves in a strange position—they've given birth, but somebody else is caring for the baby most of the time. Not only is the stress of having a sick or very small infant difficult to deal with while you're recovering from birth, but you may have felt disconnected from your baby for hours or even days after your birth if you weren't able to visit her. When you do visit, it may feel unreal that this baby was ever inside your body, and you may be afraid to touch her.

L. Essential

Many experts are now recognizing the importance of touch in helping sick and premature babies thrive. Kangaroo care, which includes holding your baby skin to skin, is an important way to help your baby get better. Kangaroo care can be done even if your baby is hooked up to wires and tubes. Visit ✍www.kangaroomothercare.com for more information.

Though nurses will probably do the majority of your baby's care at first, it's important that you do as much of her care as you're able to. Remember, while the nurses are extremely knowledgeable about caring for babies, this is your baby, and you matter to him. Instead of being intimidated and thinking of your nurse as an authority figure, think of you and your nurse as partners in helping your baby get big enough or well enough to go home with you. Ask any questions that come up, and if you need help with breastfeeding or some other aspect of baby care, ask your nurse to help you.

Going Home Without Your Baby

If your baby is in the NICU for a significant length of time after birth, you will probably be discharged before he is. It can feel very strange to go home after giving birth without a baby, almost like you never gave birth at all. Some women say that leaving their babies in the hospital while they go home is the hardest thing they've ever done, while others are surprised by how free they feel to come and go when they are "supposed" to have a baby to care for, and how they may feel guilty about that.

 Fact

Sometimes, when a mother gives birth to multiples, one baby will be discharged before the other is ready to go home. It's common for moms to feel as though they've bonded with one baby more thoroughly than the other, but with time and attention, you can become attached to both babies.

Many hospitals allow parents to visit their babies in the NICU whenever they want, except for during shift changes a few times a day. But an NICU is not the best place to get a good night's sleep, and you will need rest. Some hospitals will allow visiting moms to borrow a bed if there is room, and, as mentioned previously, others have special units set up for visiting parents. If your hospital doesn't provide beds for overnight visits from parents and you live too far away from the hospital to make the drive every day, you can find out whether there is a hospitality house or other accommodations for out-of-town guests.

Your Physical Recovery

Even though you'll probably be doing a lot of traveling back and forth from the hospital—and worrying about your baby—it is extremely important that you still care for yourself well as you're recovering from birth. Eat nutritious foods. Let your partner sit with the baby while you take a nap. Try to find some way to relax every day, since stress can make postpartum recovery more difficult.

Breastfeeding

Start pumping your breasts soon after birth and continue every few hours until your baby is able to nurse—that way, you'll be contributing in a very real and important way to your baby's care by giving him something no one else can, you'll relieve engorgement, and you'll also experience the health benefits of oxytocin. Many mothers say that when their baby was in the NICU, being cared for by doctors and nurses and surrounded by machines, pumping breastmilk was the one thing that helped them feel like their baby's mother. You can get a prescription for a breast pump from your care provider so that insurance will cover it. Get a hospital-grade electric double pump—don't skimp.

Get Help

A baby in the hospital will often mobilize friends, family, and members of your church or other organization to pitch in. Accept any help you're offered. A prayer chain; help with meals, laundry, and care of older children; and emotional support are all ways your support system can help you get through this stressful time.

Coming Home

The news that your baby is ready to leave the hospital might bring out some conflicting emotions—you'll be excited and relieved that you can finally bring him home, but also afraid that you won't know how to take care of him.

Most likely, the nurses will want to watch you with the baby to make sure you know how to care for any special needs he may have, as well as typical baby-care tasks like diapering and feeding him. Many mothers feel that they're parenting in a fishbowl, waiting for the NICU nurses to deem them worthy of the baby, but your confidence will grow with each diaper you change.

When you get home, you may find yourself ridden with anxiety about how to properly care for your baby. You may also experience a delayed reaction of mourning over the birth and new-baby experience you lost out on. This is normal. Finding a group for mothers of sick or premature babies in your area will allow you to find compassionate ears and support as you work through the feelings surrounding your baby's birth and hospitalization.

L. Essential

To spare you the stress of having to update multiple friends and family members on your baby's condition every day, consider starting a Web site or blog. Your loved ones can see pictures and read updates on your baby's progress, and you'll have a record of your baby's early weeks. Blogger is one free service; for more information, see *www.blogger.com.*

Now that your baby is home, you may feel compelled to make up for lost time by being an attentive mother 24-7. But don't neglect your own care in the process. Make sure you are eating well, showering and getting dressed daily, getting some sun and fresh air every day, and setting aside little pockets of time to yourself to recharge your batteries. Moms who've gone through the stressful experience of having a sick or premature baby are especially at risk for postpartum depression, so it's crucial that your emotional and physical needs are met during this time. Also, don't forget to communicate regularly with your partner about your feelings. You've both been through a stressful situation, and you need to keep talking to one another to keep your relationship strong.

CHAPTER 5

Recovering after a C-section

C-SECTIONS NOW ACCOUNT FOR over one quarter of all births in the United States. Far from being a minor procedure, a c-section is major abdominal surgery, and it catches many mothers by surprise. If you had your baby via c-section, you may be worried about things like breastfeeding and bonding, and you may have strong negative feelings about your surgery. This chapter will tell you how to breast-feed and bond in spite of obstacles, as well as how to take special care of yourself physically and emotionally.

Preparing for a C-section

If you're reading this while pregnant and aren't planning to have a c-section, you might think there's no reason to bother with this chapter. But while it's important to plan for the kind of birth you want, cesarean births are becoming increasingly common for a variety of reasons. In case you end up needing an emergency c-section, or your doctor just feels it's the better way to go once you're in labor, you'll want to have a good idea of what the procedure entails.

 Fact

According to the National Center for Health Statistics, over 29 per-cent of all births in the United States occurred via cesarean section in 2004. That number is expected to continue to rise.

In addition to learning the basics of the operation, it's also important to think about the kind of experience you want to have if you do end up delivering your baby via c-section. For instance, will your hospital offer you the option of watching your baby enter the world via well-placed mirrors, if you'd like to see? Will the surgeon hand you the baby so you can announce its gender and have a chance to hold him before everybody else in the room? Can you have your husband and, if possible, a doula in the operating room with you? Will you be allowed to eat after the surgery if you have a c-section? Will you be separated from your baby while you're in the recovery room, or while the surgeon is stitching you up? You'll want to consider all these factors when choosing a hospital and making your birth plan. For more information on creating a customized birth plan, see Chapter 1.

Recovering in the Hospital

You can expect your incision site to be sore for some time after your baby is born. You may want some form of pain relief, as well as additional help and support for getting around while your incision is still tender.

Pain Relief

You'll be given strong pain relief for at least the first couple of days after surgery. Your epidural or spinal block may stay in for up to a day after your c-section so that you can get more medication if you need it. Your anesthesiologist may also put morphine in your epidural, which can help with pain relief for the first day or so after surgery. Sometimes anesthesiologists will give a systemic narcotic for pain relief, or they may hook you up to a system that allows you to deliver more medication via IV when you're feeling uncomfortable. No matter what kind of pain relief you're given, be sure to ask for more if you're in pain. If you hurt, it will be harder to get started with breastfeeding, and you'll have difficulty enjoying your baby.

Effects of Medication

You may feel some aftereffects of your analgesic, such as itching, grogginess, or nausea, and your abdominal area will be sore for some time. While you're in the hospital, the staff will check your vital signs regularly, make sure that your uterus is firm, assess your bleeding, and look at your incision site to make sure it's healing properly. Anything that puts pressure on the abdominal area, like sneezing, laughing, or even moving your upper body, may hurt, especially at first. You'll need to make sure to support your incision with a hand or pillow for the first few days whenever you do anything that may strain your sutures.

Gas and Bloating

Gas and bloating are two common and uncomfortable side effects from abdominal surgery, and they plague many new moms who've delivered via c-section. Getting out of bed and moving around can help. If you're very uncomfortable, tell your nurses—they can give you an antigas medication that's safe to take while nursing.

Getting Around

Your nurses will probably encourage you to get out of bed the day of or possibly the day after surgery. Don't get out of bed by yourself the first time—you'll need a nurse to be with you in case you're shaky or dizzy. You'll want to take a few short walks, with help, each day starting the day after surgery. This will help get your digestive system moving and increase circulation, which can help you avoid developing blood clots. It may be very uncomfortable to walk at first, but keep at it; you need to move around to aid your recovery. Try timing your walks for a half hour or so after you've taken pain medication so you're experiencing its peak effectiveness. Before your first walk and while you're lying in bed during your hospital stay, you can help keep your blood circulating by moving your legs and feet.

Recovering at Home

Several days after your baby is born—usually four or so—your doctor will remove your staples or tapes. If you have sutures on the skin they will dissolve over time by themselves, and do not have to be removed. You'll be discharged. If you go home before your staples or tapes are removed (as many women do) your doctor will want you to come into his office to remove them on around day four. This can be a huge and exhausting undertaking so soon after birth and surgery. Call ahead to check that the doctor is on time with his scheduling so you won't have to wait too long. Rest before you go, and go right back home to bed. Even after you've been released from the hospital, you've still got a lot of healing to do.

How You'll Feel

Your incision will continue to be tender, and you may need to continue taking prescription pain medication for the first week or so, and then an over-the-counter drug like Tylenol or Motrin after that. You should feel a little better every day. If your incision starts to look or feel worse—swelling, oozing, or getting redder—or it feels warm, the pain gets worse, or you experience any fever, you should call your care provider right away. These could all be signs of infection.

Just like if you'd given birth vaginally, your body will discharge lochia for up to six weeks. It should go from bright red to pink or brown in the first week, and then gradually turn yellowish-white. If bright red bleeding persists past the first four days or if your bleeding turns bright red after having faded to pink or brown, call your care provider, and cut back on your activities.

Rest, Gentle Exercise, and Nutrition

You'll need to rest a lot at home, but getting up and moving around is essential to promote healing and prevent excessive gas, constipation, and other complications like blood clots. Any gas and bloating should get better as you continue to get up and move around. Don't forget to drink plenty of water and eat foods with fiber—whole grains, fruits, and vegetables—to avoid constipation.

You'll want to wait until you get clearance from your care provider before you start any kind of exercise besides gentle walking or Kegel exercises. You'll probably get the OK for pelvic tilts and other gentle abdominal exercises, but will have to hold off on crunches and more strenuous workouts. Avoid lifting anything heavier than your baby for the first six to eight weeks after delivery. After six to eight weeks, you should be feeling much better, though pain and numbness at the site of your scar may persist for some time.

Ask for Help

You're going to need help once you get home. If you're single or your partner will be returning to work shortly, ask for help from family members and friends. Paid help, if you can afford it, may be very useful. See Chapter 1 for ideas on getting help. Don't forget, your only roles right now should be caring for your baby and yourself. Housework and caring for older children should be someone else's job while you're recovering.

 Question

When will I be able to have sex again after a c-section?
You'll probably be able to resume sexual intercourse around week six, after your caregiver gives you the go-ahead. You may find that positions that put pressure on your incision site are painful or uncomfortable. Visit Chapter 16 for more tips on having an enjoyable postpartum sex life.

Your Incision Scar

Most c-section scars are horizontal and low on the abdomen, far below the waistband of your underwear or bikini bottom. Your scar will be raised, puffy, and darker than your skin at first, but will begin to shrink after a few weeks. Eventually, the scar will be very narrow (about $\frac{1}{16}$ of an inch wide), and nearly the same color as your skin.

Some women find that they have a "flap" of skin over their c-section scar. You may be able to help this flap shrink or go away with good diet and exercise, but it may stick around.

Emotional Issues after a C-section

One of the most difficult aspects of c-section recovery can be the emotional toll the surgery takes on you. If you've had a c-section, you're more likely to suffer from postpartum depression. You may feel just fine about your surgery, but you could also feel angry, sad, or guilty, and those feeling don't always come up right away.

Feeling Fine

Not every woman experiences emotional distress after a cesarean section: Some mothers feel just fine about their surgical births, or may feel relieved, especially if they were experiencing a difficult labor before the c-section, or if they or their baby had a worrisome health condition during pregnancy and the c-section resulted in a healthy mom and baby.

Negative Feelings

Many mothers grieve very deeply the loss of a vaginal birth. If you planned and prepared for a vaginal birth, you may feel cheated if things didn't go as you'd planned. If a long and difficult labor ended in c-section, you may be angry that you did all that work just to end up with a c-section in the end. You may feel that your care providers failed you, or you may feel that your body failed you. All these feelings are very normal, and you shouldn't try to "get over it." If you were planning on or hoping for a vaginal birth and ended up with a surgical birth, you have experienced a genuine loss and should be allowed to mourn that loss. You may be able to move past it quickly, or the feelings may continue to pop up for a long time. Either experience is normal—there is no time limit on the grief process.

Alert

Some women have a strong emotional reaction to their c-sections right away, but sometimes, the feelings don't pop up until weeks or months after your baby is born, when you've had time to stop and think about your birth, or you hear about a friend's birth experience.

If you don't have any negative feelings about your birth experience, it's very likely that you'll continue to feel fine with your c-section, never experiencing a sense of loss, grief, or anger. This is also normal! If you feel completely at peace with your birth, there's no need to borrow trouble by waiting on edge for the grief to kick in, or by feeling guilty because you aren't sad or disappointed by the way your birth experience played out. On the other hand, it can be helpful to know that sometimes these feelings take a while to kick in, so that you won't be taken by surprise if they do.

Talking about Your Feelings

If you're experiencing grief, anger, or other negative feelings about your c-section, it's important to talk about it with supportive people. You may even find that you have a hard time not talking about it, even if those around you aren't sure what to say or are downright dismissive of your feelings. The following sections cover the possible roadblocks you may run into when trying to express your feelings to the people in your life.

Your Spouse or Partner

While it's normal to want your partner to be your primary emotional support, your husband or partner may not be able to give you what you need when it comes to emotional support after your c-section. If you had a long or difficult labor prior to surgery, your partner may have been relieved that the surgeon took over and may not understand your sense of loss.

⌐ Essential

Men and women often have different communication styles, and it's common for men to feel the need to "fix" whatever's hurting their wives. Make sure your husband understands that you aren't asking him to solve a problem, but that you want him to simply listen with a sympathetic ear.

He may be feeling his own anxiety over the situation or may feel that it's best to put the experience behind you. Your partner may also simply not know what to do or how best to help you feel better. It's also possible that your partner will go through his own version of a grieving process later, or show it in a different way.

These differences are normal, but you can express to your partner that to heal and move past the grief you feel around your birth experience, you need to go over what happened, and you need him to offer you nonjudgmental and noncritical support.

Negative Feelings Toward Your Partner

Sometimes, difficulty in sharing your birth experience with your spouse can come from negative feelings you may be harboring toward him in connection with your birth. You may find yourself feeling angry with your partner if you feel he failed at the job of "protecting" you from the c-section. This feeling doesn't always have a basis in reality, but it can be difficult to overcome. You may also feel jealous of him if he was able to hold the baby before you were, give the baby his first feeding, or otherwise spend what you considered "your time" with the baby. Even if these feelings seem irrational, getting these feelings out is vital to moving past them—trying to squelch them will probably just lead to the feeling showing up in different ways. You can talk about them with a third party (a therapist, midwife, or doula), attend a cesarean support group, or write about these feelings in a journal. You don't necessarily have to share these feelings with your partner, but it's important to find some way to help you express them so that you can move past them.

Friends and Family

Sometimes well-meaning loved ones can actually make matters worse in their attempts to make you feel better about your birth experience. It's normal for you to want to tell your birth story again and again, but the people close to you may not understand your negative feelings—"Well, you got a healthy baby, and that's all that matters!"—or try to convince you that you "got off easy" by not giving birth vaginally. Or, your loved ones may try to convince you that you were "saved" by the c-section, which can be especially difficult to digest if you aren't entirely convinced the procedure was necessary.

Essential

If you have very different views on birth or c-sections from a friend or family member, it might not be a good idea to broach the topic with them when you're still raw from your birth. You can agree to disagree instead of causing yourself more stress with an argument.

Nowadays, surgical birth is so commonplace that many people underestimate just how big a deal it can be for a mother, and you may find yourself on the receiving end of a lot of thoughtless comments. Also, people may be so happy about your baby that they don't want to dwell on any negative feelings you might be having, and don't understand how you could be feeling sadness even when you have a new baby. On the flip side, some mothers actually report that family and friends criticize their c-section, whether it was planned or an emergency.

Your Feelings Matter

Remember, your birth experience does matter. If you feel sad, angry, disappointed, resentful, or any other negative feeling connected to your birth, it is valid. However, for a variety of reasons, including your loved ones' own fears, biases, and experiences when it comes to birth, and the cultural notion that the process of birth is not important, you may have a difficult time finding an understanding ear to listen to you express your grief over your birth experience. If your friends or family aren't able to understand your feelings surrounding your birth experience, it might be best to simply not discuss it with them, and to find an understanding person to talk it over with instead.

 Alert

If your c-section was an emergency, if you or your baby were in immediate danger of dying, if you had issues with your anesthesia that led to your feeling pain throughout the surgery, or if you had some other complication that led to an extremely stressful birth experience, you may experience what's known as posttraumatic stress disorder (PTSD). For more about PTSD, see Chapter 15.

Moving On

It can be difficult to go through a mourning process while also trying to get to know and enjoy your new baby and the experience of motherhood. While you may feel some pressure from others to "get over it" so you can focus on your baby, it's important to allow yourself your feelings. Unresolved pain can actually make it more difficult to enjoy your baby and can lead to, or worsen, depression symptoms, so allow yourself to go through this process while keeping in mind that, little by little, things will get better. There are things you can do to help yourself heal.

Tell Your Birth Story

This is a very important step in healing because it helps you define your feelings and figure out where they're coming from. This might be difficult at first. You may want to seek out an understanding person, like a member of a cesarean support group, or a professional, like a therapist or doula, so that your first experiences of telling your birth story are met with sympathy or empathy instead of judgment or criticism. You may also want to write down your birth story, perhaps submitting it to an online forum for others to read, even anonymously.

If it's hard for you to write about your birth, start small: you don't have to write the whole story at once. Start with the parts that are easiest to write or think about and work from there. You may find that you want to tell your birth story again and again, focusing on different parts. This is normal and can be a healthy way of dealing with strong feelings surrounding your birth.

Let Yourself Feel Bad

One of the most important things you can do to aid emotional healing is to simply not resist or suppress the feelings that come up when you think about your birth experience, but allow yourself to experience them. Otherwise, they will come up again and again, manifesting themselves in different ways. You may find that meditation or long walks help you tune in to the feelings and thoughts you're experiencing and help you move past them in a more healthy way.

Essential

When you're feeling badly about your birth, it can be helpful to read other mothers' stories and tell them your own. Log on to ✍www.birthstories.com to read about a variety of birth experiences, including c-sections, and maybe even share your own.

Find a Community

Tuning into a community of other women who've experienced birth-related emotional trauma can help you feel like your feelings are valid. Visit a mothering message board or check with a local hospital, birth center, or midwife's office to see if there is a support group in your area for c-section healing or birth trauma.

L. Essential

Check your local chapter of the International Cesarean Awareness Network (✎www.ican-online.com) to see if there are support groups or other resources in your area to help you recover from a c-section.

Keep a Journal

The act of getting your feelings and fears out of your head and down onto paper can be very freeing. Your journal doesn't have to be publishable or even have a beginning, middle, and end. It's for your eyes only, and can be nothing more than a random collection of doodles and scribbled words, if that's what works for you. Allow yourself to be as sad, angry, or even as mean as you want in the journal.

Bonding with Your Baby

Moms who gave birth via c-section sometimes worry that they won't bond with their babies, particularly if they didn't get to see or hold the baby for some time after delivery. Even if you were able to see your baby right after birth, medication or pain may have kept you from being able to really enjoy the experience. Some moms feel disconnected from their babies after a c-section, and may feel guilty about that.

Alert

> If you don't fall in love with your baby immediately, don't worry that it will never happen. Bonding is a process that happens over days, weeks, and months, and it's normal to feel anxiety when it comes to your baby's health. But if you have obsessive thoughts about your baby or find that you take no interest in her at all, you may be suffering from a postpartum mood disorder, and should contact your doctor or midwife, or a therapist.

On the other hand, some moms find that the c-section actually spurs them to bond even more intensely with their babies to the point that they have a hard time allowing anyone else, including their partners, to care for the baby. Either reaction is normal, and with time, moms who don't feel a connection to their babies will forge a strong attachment, while mothers who may feel anxious about ever loosening their hold on their baby will be able to relax a little.

Breastfeeding after a Cesarean

Yes, you can breastfeed after a cesarean section! A c-section birth presents a few obstacles, but they can usually be overcome. This section includes some tips and solutions to make breastfeeding as easy as possible.

Start Early

If you're feeling up to it, nursing in the recovery room immediately after surgery is the best way to get off to a good start with breastfeeding. The baby's sucking reflex is strongest in the first couple of hours after the birth, and he'll enjoy the immune-boosting benefits of colostrum (a premilk substance that is rich in antibodies and helps your baby pass his first stool). It's also good for you, helping your uterus to contract efficiently, and can help you feel more bonded to your baby, which is important if the c-section experience has left you feeling like you didn't really "give birth."

Sleepy Babies

Sometimes, babies born via c-section are a bit drowsy and lethargic because of the extended exposure to medications during labor and birth, and, if you've had little or no labor, because of the lack of stimulation a vaginal birth provides. These babies may need a little extra encouragement to stay interested and awake throughout a feeding. Or, your baby may have experienced distress or a medical condition that led to the c-section, and won't be able to nurse effectively right away. In those circumstances, your milk may take longer to come in, but you can still establish a good supply if you pump often until your baby is able to nurse, and then nurse often.

Medication Worries

The pain medication you'll receive during and after surgery should be safe for your baby to consume in the small amounts that will pass into your milk. Also, remember that in the first few days of nursing, your baby won't be getting lots of milk, but instead a small amount of colostrum. By the time your milk has come in, you'll likely be taking less medication. If you have any doubts about whether the medication the hospital staff is offering you is safe for nursing, request that they give you safe medications. It's also important that you stay comfortable so that you can get enough rest, since stress or fatigue can lead to a decreased milk supply.

Essential

> If you had a c-section, you probably received antibiotics, which can cause vaginal or nipple yeast infections, called thrush. For more information on treating thrush and preventing recurrent infections, see Chapter 8.

Positioning

If you nurse for the first time immediately after your baby is delivered, your epidural will probably still be in place. This can be a mixed blessing—it will be more comfortable to nurse while you're still numb, but you'll need to nurse lying on your back, and may have one or both arms restrained. A nurse can help position the baby and get her latched on. By the next time you breastfeed, you should have more freedom of movement, but will probably need to find positions that do not put pressure on your incision site.

L. Essential

No matter what breastfeeding position you choose, protect your incision site with a small pillow or rolled-up towel in case your baby kicks or squirms and bumps against it. You may also want to place a pillow under your knees to support your back and minimize the strain to your abdominal muscles.

Many moms who've had c-sections prefer the side-lying or football-hold position—for details on these positions, see Chapter 8. You may have to experiment a bit before you find a position that works for you and your baby. Take it slow and easy while rolling over or shifting positions in the first few days.

If you have a hard time finding a comfortable position for breast-feeding, ask a nurse for help or suggestions, or better yet, ask for a visit from the hospital's lactation consultant or breastfeeding special-ist, or call a knowledgeable friend or La Leche League volunteer.

If You and Baby Are Separated

If your baby has to spend some time in the nursery or newborn intensive care unit (NICU), you may not be able to nurse him right away. Ask for an electric breast pump and use it as soon as possible after birth and every couple of hours after that. Ask the nurses to wake you up every three to four hours to pump at night. This will help stimulate your breasts to produce milk, and even if your baby can't eat at the breast right away, your colostrum can be fed to the baby until you're able to nurse him.

If your baby can't receive your colostrum or milk right away, make sure the nurses store it properly until he can. Small or ill babies especially need the benefits of your breastmilk.

CHAPTER 6

Postpartum Complications and Health Concerns

MOST POSTPARTUM WOMEN do fine, and postpartum complications are often minor and treatable. The information in this chapter isn't meant to alarm you—serious postpartum complications are rare, especially in healthy mothers who've had normal deliveries. Still, it's important to know what's normal and what's not as you monitor your own postpartum recovery. This chapter offers a rundown of some problems—from infections to gallbladder issues—that can come up during the postpartum period.

Infections

Postpartum infections are caused by bacteria entering the uterine cavity, the urinary tract, or the site of an incision or tear. But there are also other kinds of infections that can occur during postpartum, such as breast infections and respiratory infections. Since infections can be serious, it's important to be on the lookout for fever and other signs of infection during postpartum. If you have any concerns, be sure to get in touch with your care provider immediately.

Uterine Infection

Right after you've had a baby, your body is especially vulnerable to infections of the lining of the uterus, or endometrium. If you've had a c-section, or if you've had a long labor accompanied by the early rupture of your amniotic sac, you are at a higher risk of developing a uterine infection.

Symptoms of a uterine infection include fever, lower abdominal pain, or bad-smelling lochia. If you experience any of these symptoms after you've gone home, call your doctor or midwife right away—uterine infections can be serious.

 Alert

Your uterus is usually a sterile area, but sometimes during labor and birth—particularly when there has been a lot of interference from hands or other objects in your vagina during or after labor—bacteria from your bowel, vagina, perineum, or cervix may enter the uterus and lead to an infection.

Prevention

The more hands or objects enter your vagina during labor or after birth, the more risk there is that infection-causing bacteria could be pushed upward toward your uterus. Limit internal exams during labor—some midwives and doctors don't do internal exams at all unless you ask for one—and resist the use of internal fetal monitoring, forceps, and any other procedure that would introduce an object into your vagina unless truly medically necessary. Once your baby's born, be religious about caring for your perineal area. Always use your peri bottle to rinse, wipe front to back after using the bathroom, and change your sanitary pad frequently, as pads can be a breeding ground for bacteria.

Treatment

Uterine infections can be dangerous and need to be treated with antibiotics. If it's a serious infection, you may need to be hospitalized to receive intravenous antibiotics.

If you're hospitalized for infection, you should be able to bring your baby along with you, as long as your husband or another support person is there to help you care for him. If you're nursing, be sure to ask your doctor about antibiotics that are safe for breast-feeding—they may not be part of the usual protocol, but your doctor should be able to find medications that will work for you.

Urinary Tract Infection

Sometimes bacteria from your vagina or perineum can move into your urinary tract, causing an infection that can involve just the urethra, or sometimes the bladder and kidneys, too. If you have difficulty urinating, if it hurts while you urinate (besides the initial stinging when your urine touches an abrasion, tear, or episiotomy site), or if your urine is cloudy, dark, scanty, or bloody, it could be that you've got a UTI. Other symptoms include fever, chills, pain in your back or side, and feelings like you have to go to the bathroom all the time, but then little or nothing actually comes out.

Prevention

Frequent trips to the bathroom and drinking enough water are crucial to keeping your urinary tract healthy. Again, using your peri bottle, wiping from front to back after using the bathroom, and frequently changing your sanitary pad will help keep bacteria from your vagina and anus from entering your urethra. If you had an epidural during labor or had trouble urinating afterward, you may have had a catheter inserted, which also raises the risk of UTIs. Unsweetened cranberry juice and cranberry pills have both been shown to help prevent UTIs.

Treatment

Your treatment will depend on how far into your urinary tract the infection has moved. You'll probably be given antibiotics, and depending on how serious the infection, they may need to be given intravenously. You'll be told to drink a lot of water to flush the bacteria out of your urinary tract, and your urine will usually be tested at the beginning and end of the treatment to see how the medication worked.

Incision, Episiotomy, or Tear Site Infection

Incision sites from a c-section or episiotomy are susceptible to infection. If you notice redness, tenderness, or discharge from or swelling around the site of a wound, it could indicate an infection.

Prevention

Avoid an episiotomy if you can. Many experts now agree that routine episiotomy is not justified, and the deep, intramuscular wounds they create can become infected. Pushing gently, with your body's signals, and in the position of your choice, instead of forced "purple-faced" pushing can help you avoid or reduce tearing and lessen the chances of this type of infection. If you've had a c-section, keep your stitches dry and clean. For both tears and episiotomies, follow the infection-fighting rules of peri care, wiping front to back, and changing your sanitary pad often.

Treatment

Sometimes, the sutures at an infected incision site will have to be opened and the wound drained and restitched. You'll probably receive a local anesthetic, similar to the one you received when it was originally stitched, for this procedure. You may also be given antibiotics, depending on how serious the infection is. Remember to ask your doctor for antibiotics that are safe for breastfeeding.

Breast Infection

Engorgement, cracked nipples, and clogged ducts, which are common in the early days of breastfeeding, can lead to mastitis, or breast infections. If you feel like you're getting the flu, with fever or chills, muscle aches, or fatigue, and these symptoms are coupled with a painful, swollen, red, hard area or red streaks on the breast that may feel warm to the touch, you probably have a breast infection.

Fact

Giving birth in water is a growing trend in the United States and has been linked with fewer and less severe perineal tearing during pushing. Some experts feel that warm water helps the perineal tissues open and stretch, while others hypothesize that the slow, low-intervention nature of water birth means fewer hands and objects in the way that could cause tearing. Being able to move about freely and adjust instinctively to your baby's descent and emergence also helps.

Prevention

Avoid underwire bras or anything that's tight on your breasts (if it leaves marks, that's a good indicator that it's too tight). If you start to feel under the weather, go to bed, nurse often, drink plenty of fluids, and rest.

Treatment

If you develop mastitis, drink lots of fluids, eat nutritious food, and rest, rest, rest. Tylenol or Motrin can help relieve discomfort and bring fever down, and vitamin C may help boost your immunity to help you fight off the infection. Use heat to keep the ducts open, and massage your breasts to keep the milk flowing. Some doctors advise women to wean if they develop mastitis. This is not necessary and can actually make things worse! If your care provider prescribes an antibiotic, insist on a breastfeeding-friendly one.

Hemorrhage

It's normal to lose some blood after giving birth. When the placenta separates from the uterine wall, the resulting wound bleeds until the blood vessels close off with help from your contracting uterus. And since your body's blood volume increases by about 50 percent during pregnancy, some blood loss won't affect your health.

But sometimes, women bleed too much after giving birth, which is called a postpartum hemorrhage. This happens in up to 5 percent of all births, and is most likely to happen while the placenta is separating or soon afterward.

 Alert

Sometimes, a mother will hemorrhage days or even weeks after birth. This rare but serious condition is called a late or delayed postpartum hemorrhage and is usually caused by retained membranes or tissue in the uterus. If you experience unexpected heavy bleeding days or weeks postpartum, lie down, stay warm, nurse your baby if possible, and call 911.

A few things can make it more likely that you'll bleed too much after giving birth. One cause of postpartum hemorrhage (PPH) is called uterine atony, which means that your uterus has difficulty contracting effectively after birth because it's been overstretched or is tired out. If your labor was induced or augmented with pitocin, you're more likely to experience postpartum hemorrhage. Also, if your uterus was stretched due to an overabundance of amniotic fluid or because you were pregnant with multiples, or if your uterus tired out due to a very long or very short labor, you may be at a higher risk of postpartum hemorrhage.

Another cause of PPH is when your placenta doesn't separate from the uterus quickly enough, or only separates partially, leaving behind exposed blood vessels. This is most often caused by someone pulling on the cord or massaging the uterus too roughly. Uterine fibroids, large blood clots, or fragments of placenta left behind can also make it difficult for your uterus to contract effectively.

Essential

> A condition called placenta accreta, when the placenta is implanted too deeply in the uterus and can't separate, can also cause postpartum hemorrhage. The risk of placenta accreta grows with each c-section you have. Placenta accreta is diagnosed shortly after birth and is rare but serious.

Episiotomies or tears in your cervix, vagina, or perineum can also cause some postpartum bleeding. Generally, the amount of bleeding from a tear or episiotomy isn't something to be worried about, but if the episiotomy is large or you have deep or extensive tears, you could lose a considerable amount of blood.

Women with blood-clotting disorders—which can be due to a pregnancy-related condition like pre-eclampsia or a placental abruption—are more likely to bleed heavily. And very rarely, a ruptured or inverted uterus can cause hemorrhage.

Prevention

Like other postpartum complications, your care provider and birth experience can have a significant impact on how much you'll bleed after giving birth. Frequent trips to the bathroom and breastfeeding early and often can help your uterus contract effectively and limit bleeding.

Treatment

If you're bleeding too much after giving birth, your care provider will first determine where the bleeding is coming from. You'll be given an IV to keep your blood pressure up. If the bleeding is coming from an episiotomy or tear, your doctor or midwife will stitch it, and that should stop the bleeding. If the bleeding is coming from your uterus and your placenta has not yet come out, your doctor or midwife may have to manually remove it, or he or she may have to remove blood clots or retained placenta fragments. You may receive a shot or an IV of oxytocin, and your caregiver will massage your uterus to help it contract. Your caregiver may need to massage your uterus directly, with one hand on your belly and one hand inside your vagina.

 Question

I've heard that some women require a dilation and curettage (D&C) after giving birth. Could this happen to me?
If your doctor or midwife is unable to get placenta fragments out any other way, a D&C, abdominal surgery, or even a hysterectomy could be required. It's extremely rare, though, and it's very unlikely that it will happen to you.

During the time that your care provider is assessing and treating the bleeding, your blood pressure and pulse will be monitored to give signs as to how you're coping with blood loss.

Recovery after Hemorrhage

If you hemorrhage, you'll continue to receive IV fluids and medication to help your uterus stay contracted after the bleeding is under control, and you'll be watched closely for further bleeding. How long it takes to recover and how you'll feel afterward will depend on how much blood you lost, how much your blood volume increased during your pregnancy, and whether or not you were anemic. You may feel dizzy, weak, or lightheaded, and you'll need help getting out of bed. Be sure to get lots of rest, drink plenty of fluids, and eat nutritious food. You may want to take an iron supplement. Floradix is a good choice: it's a food-based iron supplement that's well absorbed by your body and won't cause constipation. Rarely, blood transfusions may be necessary after a hemorrhage.

Hematoma

A hematoma occurs when blood collects in the tissues that stretch and open while your baby is being born, creating a painful, sometimes large lump or swollen spot in the perineal area. Hematomas are usually caused by the pressure of pushing your baby out, or by an imperfect stitching job in which the two sides of the skin are not completely closed together. Though the bleeding below the skin or mucus membranes usually stops on its own, the pooled blood can be prone to infection and can also lead to a longer healing period for the perineal area, so a hematoma should be reported to your health-care provider immediately.

Essential

Many midwives swear by homeopathic Arnica for treatment of postpartum bruising, tissue trauma, and soreness. Arnica comes in pellet, gel, and cream form and can be found in many drugstores and health-food stores. Don't use cream or gel on broken skin, and be sure to get the homeopathic version of the pills, which are considered safe for nursing mothers.

If a hematoma becomes infected, it can cause the edges of a tear or episiotomy repair to pull apart from one another, and they may not be able to re-adhere. If this happens, you may have to return to the hospital for repair, and there can be significant blood loss and pain.

Prevention

The use of forceps during birth; rough handling of your uterus, vaginal area, or perineum during labor, birth, or postpartum; or a mismanaged repair job can all increase the risk of hematomas. Again, the rules seem to be that the more gently you are treated during labor and birth, the better your postpartum recovery will be.

Treatment

Your midwife or doctor will prescribe antibiotics and may also advise alternating hot and cold soaks. The heat will stimulate circulation, while the cold can decrease swelling and relieve pain. Your care provider may also recommend a rinse of warm water with a bit of antiseptic after using the toilet, and you'll want to gently and thoroughly pat your perineal area dry or allow it to air dry after each trip to the bathroom.

Bruised, Sprained, or Broken Tailbone

If you feel pain at the base of your spine, near your coccyx (tailbone), you may have broken or bruised your tailbone or sprained the joint between your coccyx and sacrum during labor and birth. While there isn't necessarily a quick fix here, it's still important that you recognize the problem and allow for it to heal.

Prevention

Tailbone injuries can be caused by several factors, but the only one you have any real control over is your baby's position. If your baby's head is bumping up against your tailbone during labor and delivery, it can cause injury and pain. See Chapter 1 for information on how your baby's position can affect your birth and postpartum experience, and how you can help him settle into a place that's comfortable and healthy for both of you.

Treatment

There's no real way to stabilize a broken tailbone (you can't put a cast on it), so the best thing you can do is take it easy and wait for it to heal on its own, which may take months.

It might hurt to sit or put pressure on the tailbone, so try sitting on a ring-shaped pillow (the same kind recommended for women with hemorrhoids) or a Boppy nursing pillow. Lying on your side will probably be more comfortable. Alternating heating pads or warm baths with an ice pack on the sore area can aid healing and reduce pain and swelling, and the pain should go away completely within a couple of months. If the pain is still acute after the first week, let your caregiver know. He or she may recommend massage, or a visit to a chiropractor or an osteopath for spinal manipulation to speed healing and relieve some of the pain.

 Question

What is pubic separation?
Sometimes the pubic cartilage separates before or during birth. This can range from very uncomfortable to debilitating. To help it heal, keep your legs close together when lifting or moving, and try a hip belt for stabilization. An adjustment from an osteopathic doctor (DO) or chiropractor may be able to help relieve pain and assist your body in healing itself.

Pelvic Floor Injury

Pressure from pregnancy, labor, and birth can cause your pelvic floor—the muscles, ligaments, and connective tissue of your pelvis that support your bladder, uterus, and rectum—to become weak or stretched out. This can cause prolapse, or dropping, of the organs and tissue in the pelvic area. Symptoms tend to occur when the woman is upright and to disappear when she is lying down. For some women, sexual intercourse is painful. Mild cases may not cause symptoms until a woman is older.

Conditions caused by a pelvic floor injury include:

- **Rectocele.** This occurs when the rectum protrudes into the back wall of the vagina. It can make it difficult to have a bowel movement or cause a feeling of constipation. Some women need to apply perineal or vaginal pressure in order to have a bowel movement.

- **Enterocele.** This happens when the small intestine and lining of the abdominal cavity sag down between the uterus and rectum and can cause a sense of fullness, pressure, or pain in the pelvis or lower back.
- **Cystocele.** This occurs when the bladder protrudes into the front wall of the vagina and can cause stress incontinence (urine leakage during coughing, laughing, or sneezing), or it can cause you to leak urine if your bladder becomes too full. It can also be difficult to feel that your bladder is empty, and increases the chances that you'll develop a bladder infection.
- **Uterine prolapse.** This is when the uterus sags down into the vagina. It can cause pain in the lower back or over the tailbone, or if the prolapse is severe, pain during walking, difficulty with urination or bowel movements, or bleeding sores on the cervix.

Prevention

Kegel exercises help keep the pelvic floor strong and can help prevent or treat pelvic-floor injuries. Also, maintaining a healthy weight during and after pregnancy can reduce stress and strain on the pelvic floor and reduce the chances of this type of injury. During birth, fundal pressure, which is when a caregiver pushes on your uterus to move the baby down the birth canal; forceps or vacuum extraction; giving birth lying flat on your back; or coached pushing, as opposed to pushing when you feel the urge, can all increase the chances that you'll experience a pelvic-floor injury.

Treatment

Kegel. Kegel, Kegel. For severe injuries, a device called a pessary may be used to support the pelvic organs. Estrogen suppositories or cream are another potential treatment. In some cases, surgery may be needed, but usually this won't happen until you've decided not to have any more children.

L. Essential

Remember how to do a Kegel exercise? It's so important that the directions bear repeating: Gently tighten your perineal muscles as if you were trying to stop urinating. Slowly pull the muscles up as tightly as you can—it may help to visualize an elevator going up a shaft—hold for a few seconds, and slowly release. Repeat often.

Gallbladder Issues

While it's not necessarily considered to be a complication of childbirth, gallbladder problems can be more common in the days, weeks, and months after having a baby because of hormonal changes that go along with the pregnancy and postpartum period.

The gallbladder stores bile, which helps your body digest fat. High levels of estrogen and progesterone, produced in abundance during pregnancy, can keep the gallbladder from contracting, slow the process of emptying bile from the gallbladder, and can cause gallstones.

An estimated 12 percent of pregnant women develop gallstones, which can necessitate surgery to remove the gallbladder. A gallbladder "attack" can be extremely painful. You would feel it in the upper abdomen, in the back between your shoulder blades, or under your right shoulder. You might also experience nausea, vomiting, or abdominal bloating. The symptoms are often worse or most noticeable after eating a fatty meal.

Prevention

Maintain a healthy weight and eat a high-fiber diet that's reasonably low in fat and cholesterol, and high in antioxidants. Losing or gaining weight too quickly can contribute to gallbladder problems, so take it easy with postpartum weight loss—no more than a pound or two per week. Drink lots of fluids, especially water. Dandelion tea is excellent for nourishing the gallbladder. Also, exercise during pregnancy and, as soon as you're healed enough, postpartum: one study indicated that exercising five times per week for thirty minutes could lead to a one-third reduction in the risk of developing gallstones.

Treatment

Your doctor may recommend medication to break up gallstones. In some instances, surgery will be needed. There are also alternative treatments for gallbladder problems that may work for you. Consult with a naturopath or herbalist if this approach appeals to you. If you experience any of the following symptoms: nausea, vomiting, pain in your upper abdomen, pain between your shoulder blades, or pain under your right shoulder, call your care provider.

Tips for a Healthy Postpartum Period

There are some things you can do to avoid postpartum complications and health problems. Before your baby is born, eat a healthy diet that's high in leafy green vegetables, red meat, or legumes to avoid iron-deficiency anemia. Generally you'll have blood tests late in your pregnancy to test for iron levels, and if you're anemic, you can start treatment with iron-rich foods and supplements. Perform Kegel exercises daily, as described in Chapter 3, to help keep your pelvic-floor muscles strong.

Choose Your Care Providers Carefully

Many of the conditions considered to be postpartum complications actually start with, or can be caused by, what happens during your labor and birth. When you're considering whether to use pain medication, or whether to allow a certain procedure or intervention during your labor and birth, keep in mind not only its effects on your baby and birth experience, but also what it might mean for your postpartum experience. You'll want to be sure to talk to your doctor or midwife before your birth to find out how he or she feels about things like routine interventions and c-sections. There's more information on how your birth can affect your postpartum experience—and how to choose a postpartum-friendly care provider and hospital or birthing center—in Chapter 1.

 Alert

> Call 911 or your local emergency number any time you experience the following during postpartum: shortness of breath, chest pain, coughing up blood, profuse bleeding, or the signs of shock (rapid or irregular heartbeat, shallow or rapid breathing, disorientation, clammy skin, extreme weakness, dizziness, or light-headedness).

Take It Easy

After you've given birth, take it easy, resting as much as possible for at least the first seven to ten days postpartum. During the immediate postpartum period, high levels of oxytocin in your blood are helping your uterus return to its prepregnant size. Stress creates adrenaline, which can make it more difficult for the hormones to do their job. Stay in bed and let your partner or a friend or relative (or paid help, if necessary) care for you. Be religious about caring for your perineum. Breastfeed your baby often to keep your uterus firm and limit bleeding. Eat nutritious foods and drink plenty of water. Don't lift anything heavier than your baby, and just try to rest and relax as much as you can. Limit visitors.

When to Call Your Doctor or Midwife

No matter how good you may be feeling otherwise, there are some instances when you shouldn't hesitate to call your health-care provider. Seemingly normal conditions like soreness or a headache can become serious causes for concern if they persist or worsen. Consider the following points:

- If bleeding doesn't taper off, continues to be bright red after the first four days, soaks a pad every hour, or smells bad, let your doctor or midwife know. Some large clots are normal in the first couple of days after giving birth and aren't a reason for concern as long as you aren't bleeding heavily. These large clots are caused by blood pooling and clotting in your vagina while you are lying down or sitting, and will fall out when you get up or go to the bathroom.

- If you develop a fever, even a low-grade one, tell your doctor or midwife. "Milk fever" isn't too uncommon on about day two or three postpartum or when your breasts are engorged. Still, it's best to let your care provider know what's going on. If you have no other symptoms and your care provider suspects that your fever is due to breast engorgement, he or she may tell you to try lots of water and rest before moving on to other treatment.

- If you have severe pain in your abdomen or pelvis or if your afterpains get worse after you've gone home, or if your pain or soreness gets worse or lasts beyond the first week or two, let your doctor or midwife know.

- If you have swelling, discharge, increasing pain or redness at the site of your episiotomy, tear, IV needle, or c-section incision, it could indicate infection. Call your doctor or midwife.

- If your breasts are sore, tender, red, or warm to the touch and the symptoms are not relieved by nursing, massage, and soaks in a hot tub or shower, it could indicate a breast infection, particularly if the symptoms are accompanied by fever, chills, muscle aches, or fatigue. Let your doctor or midwife know.

- If it burns or hurts when you urinate, if you feel like you have to go to the bathroom frequently but nothing or very little comes out, or if your urine is dark, cloudy, or bloody, it could indicate a urinary tract infection. Call your doctor or midwife. You may experience some stinging after the urine comes out from an abrasion or tear, and that's normal.

- If you experience severe vomiting, contact your care provider immediately.
- If you have severe or persistent headaches, double vision, blurred or dim vision, or see flashing spots or lights, let your care provider know. This could indicate a rare condition called postpartum pre-eclampsia, dangerously high blood pressure after giving birth.
- If you experience pain, tenderness, and warmth in one leg, or if one leg is more swollen than the other, it could indicate deep vein thrombosis, a blood clot. This is serious—don't hesitate to call your doctor or midwife if you have this symptom!

Many new mothers have the tendency to focus all their attention on their new baby, which, in some respects, is as it should be. However, if you're feeling ill or are in pain, you won't be able to give your baby the complete care and attention she needs. Don't wait until a small problem has escalated into a full-fledged health emergency. Accept help from family and friends, keep your care provider in the loop, and listen to all the messages your body sends you, no matter how small.

CHAPTER 7

Weeks Two to Six

AFTER THE FIRST FEW exciting and confusing days after your baby is born are over, you will probably be looking forward to that six-week mark, when most women get the green light for everything from sex to exercise. The first six weeks can be emotional, exciting, and exhausting, and you may wonder just how long it'll take to feel and look like yourself again. But remember that your baby will never be so new again. Cut yourself plenty of slack, and try to enjoy this very special time with your new baby.

How You'll Be Feeling

During the second week postpartum, many women feel a burst of energy and may seem more like normal. Enjoy this boost, but remember that you still have healing to do and need to take it easy. Your body will probably still be showing aftereffects of the birth, so you'll have to make sure you don't do too much too quickly and undo the healing you've already accomplished.

Bleeding

Your lochia should continue to taper off over the first six weeks postpartum. However, there's no definite timetable for how long it will take for this transition to happen.

To handle bleeding during the first few weeks postpartum, you can wear menstrual pads, just like you would during your period. Some women prefer cloth menstrual pads because they're softer and more breathable and they don't chafe. You can make them yourself from cotton flannel, or purchase them through catalogs or Web sites carrying eco-friendly products. You may also be able to find them at your local health-food or natural-products store. As mentioned previously, do not use tampons during the first six weeks postpartum. They can harbor bacteria, and during this time your pelvic area is particularly vulnerable to infection.

 Fact

> Postpartum bleeding doesn't always follow a textbook pattern. Sometimes it can take longer for bleeding to stop with second and subsequent pregnancies, and what's typical for another woman may not be typical for you. As long as the flow is decreasing, not increasing, and isn't going back to bright red, it's probably your body's version of normal.

You should call your care provider if you pass large blood clots after the first week postpartum. If your bleeding has turned brown or white but returns to red, it's probably a sign you've been doing too much. Check with your doctor or midwife just to be on the safe side—he or she will probably tell you to slow down and rest. Still, you'll want to let them know it's happening, so that they can rule out infection or other possible causes.

Breasts

You'll probably be getting the hang of breastfeeding by now. Your engorgement will pass, and your breasts will probably leak less and begin to regulate their milk production to make only as much as your baby will need. If your nipples are still sore, there may be something going on besides run-of-the-mill tenderness. Check out Chapter 8 to troubleshoot possible problems.

Soreness and Stitches

Any stitches or tears should be well on their way to healing by this point, though you may still notice some tenderness or soreness in your perineum, particularly at the end of the day when you're tired or have been standing a lot. Rest, keep doing your Kegel exercises regularly to keep the blood circulating in this area, and continue using your peri bottle when you go to the bathroom, as long as it feels like it's helping.

Your Pelvic Floor

In Chapter 6 you read about pelvic-floor injuries like uterine and bladder prolapse. You're at most risk for developing these conditions in the first six weeks postpartum, and too-strenuous exercise and activity greatly increases your risk. Don't overdo it! Even if you get a bolt of energy and feel like you can jump right back into all your old household chores, you're still healing and need to take it easy.

Hemorrhoids

If you developed hemorrhoids during pregnancy or birth, they may still be sore or itchy a few weeks after birth. But your hemorrhoids should begin to shrink and feel less painful during this time. If they continue to bleed or remain very sore, you'll want to talk to your doctor or midwife about them.

 Fact

Certain nutrients are linked with increased vein health, and consuming more of them may aid in healing hemorrhoids and preventing them from becoming an issue in the future. Vitamin C, bioflavinoids, vitamin E, and essential fatty acids are all vital to vein health. These nutrients are most effective when consumed as part of a healthy diet containing dark green leafy vegetables, citrus fruits and berries, and healthy fats like the kind found in fish, flaxseed, and olive oil.

Sometimes, hemorrhoids are a big enough problem that they have to be removed. Be vigilant about helping your hemorrhoids heal; continue to eat enough fiber and drink plenty of fluids. Caffeine, which is found in chocolate, coffee, tea, and soda, can be constipating and may make hemorrhoids worse. If you suffer from hemorrhoids, it's best to avoid or cut back on caffeine.

Also, instead of wiping with toilet paper, you can try flushable wet wipes medicated with witch hazel, available at drugstores. Or, you can continue to use your peri bottle for cleansing the area after using the bathroom, and just pat dry with soft toilet paper.

Even if you can't feel your hemorrhoids anymore, it doesn't mean they're not there. Once the vein wall is weakened, you'll be prone to developing hemorrhoids in the future. Be sure to always drink enough water and eat enough fiber to keep your stools soft and regular, and don't strain while having a bowel movement.

L. Essential

You may have developed varicose veins in your legs or vulva during pregnancy. Since a hemorrhoid is basically a varicose vein in the rectum, some of the same advice applies for soothing and shrinking these swollen blood vessels: consume plenty of vein-strengthening nutrients, keep your blood circulating, and elevate the affected area whenever possible.

Hemorrhoids can also be caused or worsened by too much sitting, standing, or inactivity. You shouldn't overdo it in the first six weeks postpartum, but changing positions often and going for gentle strolls around the house or block can keep your blood moving.

Also, assuming a knee-chest position—from your hands and knees, bend forward so that your rear end is sticking up and your chest is resting on the bed—every once in a while can take the pressure off the veins in your bottom. Avoid chairs that create a V in which the lowest point is your perineum, like recliners.

How You'll Look

During weeks two to six, your body will slowly start to return closer to prepregnant shape. Don't expect to have your prepregnancy body back by week three; this is a slow process. Still, chances are that you will start dropping weight, your figure will begin to reveal itself, and you'll begin to look more like your old self. The not-so-good news is that certain changes—like some loose skin on your belly or wider hips—may be here to stay.

Your Shape

Though your stomach will continue to shrink, you probably won't be back in your prepregnancy wardrobe yet. Many women find that they need to wear maternity clothes or larger sizes, with elastic-waist or drawstring pants, for weeks after they give birth. You may notice that the skin on your belly seems stretched out; it may even hang down when you stand or lie on your side. This is normal. Mothers' bodies rarely look like the airbrushed perfection seen on celebrity moms on the covers of magazines. Over time, your skin will tighten, stretch marks will fade, and your shape will begin to look more like it did before you got pregnant, but you may always carry changes as a reminder of your pregnancy.

Weight

You'll continue to lose weight as the excess fluids and fat your body stored during pregnancy are eliminated, but it's going to be a while before you're back to your prepregnancy weight. Keep in mind that during pregnancy your body may have changed permanently; you may look better at a slightly higher weight with your new structure and shape. For more information on postpartum weight loss, see Chapter 13.

Question

How much weight should I lose in the first few weeks postpartum?
It's important for your health that you don't lose weight too quickly—after the initial drop, one or two pounds per week should be your maximum goal. Remember, it took you nine months to gain your pregnancy weight, and you should give yourself at least that long to take it off.

Breast Size

Now that your breasts aren't so engorged, they may be the same size they were prepregnancy, bigger, or even smaller. You'll probably continue to notice some changes over the next few months, especially if you start breastfeeding less or wean your baby, but this is a good time to get a few bras in the size you're currently wearing.

Posture

After a few weeks of nursing and holding an infant much of the day, many women begin to adopt some bad habits when it comes to posture. You may find that you're slouching or hunching your shoulders over, or that you overcompensate by becoming somewhat swaybacked. In Chapter 12, you'll learn about some exercises you can do to improve your postpartum posture.

Getting Out of the House

Chances are, you'll eventually start to feel bored by staying at home and will want to consider venturing out for a shopping trip or a meal in a restaurant. This is a good thing; a change of scenery will reinvigorate you. It's important to realize, however, that a trip to the grocery store or a walk around the neighborhood is not going to be as simple as you remember it. For one thing, those first few trips outside the house may tire you and your baby out. Make your trips short and close by, and plan for a friend or your partner to go with you.

How Your Baby Will React

Some babies do just fine with these early trips, but some react with fussiness or sleeplessness to the unfamiliar smells and sounds and the disruption of the routine they've become accustomed to. Don't plan too much running around in these early weeks, and give yourself plenty of time in between outings to rest and relax.

Let friends or family know that you may have to cancel your plans if you don't feel up to it or if your baby isn't coping well. As you feel stronger and your baby gets older, outings will become easier to manage.

Carrying Your Baby

Using a sling or baby carrier is a great way to keep your baby close by you while you're out and about. Your baby will be comforted by your familiar smells, the sound of your heartbeat, and your warmth, even as she's being surrounded by a new world of experiences. It's very easy for a baby to become overstimulated, and this is one way to protect her from taking in too much too fast. If you wear your baby on your chest, she can always snuggle her face into the familiar scent and feel of you if the world around her becomes too much to handle.

You've probably noticed parents lugging their babies around in bucket-style infant car seats to and from the car, or even through a store or restaurant. These seats are nice because they do double duty: They function as both car seat and carrier. On the other hand, infant car seats are heavy, bulky, and awkward, and not really designed to be carried long distances. Carrying one all over can strain your arm and shoulder and leave your legs bruised. Unless you have some other reason for needing to take the car seat with you, leave it in the car and carry your baby to and from your vehicle in your arms or in a sling or baby carrier.

Consider the Details

Take the weather, time of day, and where you'll be going into account as you make your plans. If it's very hot or cold, your baby's immature nervous system may make it hard for her to regulate her body temperature. If you're heading to a very bright or noisy location, your baby may become overstimulated and either "check out" by falling into a deep sleep or become anxious and fussy. Also keep in mind that your baby's young lungs won't be able to handle environmental toxins like car exhaust or pesticides as well as most adults'. Take things like smog, ozone levels, and potential pollutants into account when taking a young baby out on the town.

Nursing in Public

Sooner or later, every nursing mom is faced with a room full of people and a hungry baby. Learning to nurse in public in a way you're comfortable with will make breastfeeding even more easy and convenient.

That's What Breasts Are For

It's natural to feel uncomfortable the first few times you nurse your baby in public. Breasts have been so sexualized in this culture that a lot of people forget that our breasts' primary function is to nourish babies.

But there's a lot of hypocrisy involved in the idea that nursing publicly is indecent. Think about it: How often do you get through an entire day without seeing almost-exposed breasts, whether they're on a magazine cover or popping out of a low-cut shirt on a girl at the mall? Most nursing mothers show far less skin than that while nursing their babies. It takes just a moment to get the baby latched on, which you can do turned away from the action in the room. Once he's latched on, your baby's head will cover your nipple and all or most of your breast.

You're Within Your Rights

Breastfeeding in public is legal anywhere in the United States. Some states have laws specifically reinforcing and protecting a mother's right to breastfeed her baby in any public place, while other states have legislated that breastfeeding does not constitute indecent exposure. Unfortunately, many people are still ignorant of this, and nursing mothers are sometimes harassed by security guards or other authority figures who don't know any better. If anyone asks you to move to a private area or, worse yet, the bathroom (would *you* eat your dinner in a restroom?) while nursing, you can calmly tell them that you are within your rights to nurse anywhere you and your baby are allowed to be together. If they persist, ask to speak to their supervisor. No one should make you feel uncomfortable about feeding your baby when he's hungry.

⌐ Essential

If you have very large breasts, you may have to be creative about nursing in public. For instance, you might have a hard time finding nursing bras and clothing in your size, or it may be more difficult to nurse discreetly. Keep practicing. As you get more comfortable with nursing in general, you'll probably become less concerned with the possibility that somebody might see a flash of skin.

Practice Makes Perfect

Regardless of their right to nurse in public, many women are a little timid about actually doing it. If you are nervous about taking your show on the road without rehearsing first, practice a few times in front of a full-length mirror, either at home or in a dressing room in a department or clothing store. You will probably be surprised by how little—if any—skin actually shows while you're nursing your baby, especially if you're wearing a loose-fitting shirt or nursing top.

Find a Quiet Spot

A comfortable chair or bench that's a little bit out of the way makes an easier, more relaxing way to ease into breastfeeding in public. Some babies are very distracted by bright lights, noises, and people walking by. The first time you nurse in public, try bringing a friend or your husband along to sit next to you and give you a hand getting the baby latched on and your clothing settled back into place. Having another person there can help you feel less exposed.

L. Essential

If you aren't comfortable with breastfeeding right out in the open at first, try nursing in your car, a dressing room, a corner booth at a restaurant, or even in the outdoor furniture section at the department store. As your baby gets older, nursing gets easier, and you're out and about more, you'll figure out the techniques and places that work best for you.

Try a Sling

Baby slings make it easy to nurse in public discreetly. They cover you up and leave both your hands free for getting positioned—you can just tuck your baby's face down into the sling over your breast and lift your shirt. It can be tricky to nurse in a sling the first few times, so practice at home, or better yet, ask the person who sold you the sling or a knowledgeable friend to help you get the hang of it.

To Cover Up or Not?

Some moms prefer to cover up with a blanket or shawl when nursing, but this method has some distinct disadvantages:

- A blanket can block your view of your baby entirely, making it much trickier to get him latched on just right.

- Your baby might get too hot underneath a blanket or shawl, or he may not like being unable to see you and may refuse to nurse.
- Covering up announces to the world: Hey! There's some breastfeeding going on under here! It may make it more obvious that you're nursing.
- Instead of putting a blanket all the way over the baby's head and shoulder, you might consider just wrapping it around his body, coming up a little behind his head. That way you can cover any part of your stomach or side that might be exposed, and his head will get a little bit of cover without being too hot or stuffy.

If you're covering up to avoid offending people, you're doing it for the wrong reasons. Breastfeeding is natural, and it's healthy for both you and your baby. Ignore the strange looks and whispers, and do whatever you think is best.

When Your Partner Returns to Work

At some point during this time, your partner or husband will probably go back to work, and you'll be left alone at home with the baby for a large part of the day. It can be difficult to make this transition, especially if you have older children in the house, aren't quite feeling up to caring for the baby by yourself, or are craving social connections but all your friends are at work during the day.

Remember to Care for Yourself

"I don't even have time to take a shower!"—it's a common refrain among new moms. But it's important to remember that you can't take good care of your baby unless you're caring for yourself, too. It is important to be flexible with your standards instead of simply sticking to your old schedule, but don't neglect those things that help you feel like a fully functional human being. Make a short list of the things you feel like you absolutely must do every day to help you feel like yourself. Reading the paper? Listening to music? Those things can be incorporated into life with a new baby.

For many women, that all-important daily shower is their personal normalcy benchmark: Get one, and life seems manageable; miss it, and everything feels "off." Here are some creative ways to get in a shower if you don't have a spouse or partner around to hold your baby:

- Set up a bouncy seat or Moses basket for your baby on the bathroom floor. Many babies are comforted by the background noise of the shower and bathroom fan, perhaps long enough to get you a nice shower.
- Take your baby into the shower with you. There are mesh shower slings, made for just this purpose.
- Try taking your baby into the bathroom in just her diaper, and starting your shower alone. Wash your hair first. Then, if the baby starts to lose it and you aren't quite done yet, you can quickly strip her naked, pop her into a mesh sling, and finish the shower that way, or let the tub fill and relax in the bath together. If you do this, have a towel on the floor next to the bathtub—then you can wrap her up in it and lay her next to the tub while you get out safely yourself.

Caring for Your Appearance

It's important that you stick to some kind of personal-care routine during this time. It doesn't have to mean putting on a full face of makeup or getting dressed in a business suit, but brushing your hair and teeth and staying clean is an essential way to keep your sense of well-being intact.

Even if you're just putting on a new pair of pajamas, sweats, or yoga pants, changing into fresh, clean clothes when you get up in the morning is one of those reminders that your day has begun and you're a part of it.

Keep your wardrobe simple and comfortable during this time. Choose clothes that are breathable, loose enough not to bind your stomach or breasts, and easy to nurse in. For more tips on choosing a postpartum wardrobe, see Chapter 14.

Older Children

If you have other children, you may find yourself torn between meeting the many needs of your new baby and giving your older kids attention and love, too. An older child may feel jealous of the new baby, too, which may make him clingier—and you may wonder if you'll ever be able to handle caring for them both! Here are a few ways you can help your older child feel special and included while keeping your sanity intact:

- Present your older child with a "big brother" or "big sister" gift after your baby is born.
- Ask grandparents, aunts, uncles, or friends to call and ask specifically to talk with your older child. Remind them to talk to the child as an individual, not just as the baby's big brother or sister.
- Try to make nursing sessions special for your older child, too. With some practice, you can juggle nursing with reading a book or snuggling an older child on the couch. When you're still getting the hang of nursing and need both hands, you can listen to stories on tape, make up a story, or tell one from memory—or ask your older child to tell *you* a story.
- Try to involve your older children in your baby's care. Even toddlers can "help" with diaper or clothing changes or apply lotion to your baby's legs (though it's probably a good idea to keep little fingers away from the baby's eyes).
- Your partner can take your older children along on errands for some one-on-one daddy time.

As your baby gets older and you feel up to it, you'll be able to spend more one-on-one time with older children, too. In the meantime, don't worry too much that your older child will be neglected—just try to spend some time cuddling and talking every day, and remember that the newborn period will go by quickly for all of you. Also, see Chapter 1 for ways to make sure you are getting enough help with your older children.

Remember to Eat

It's easy to drop meals in these early weeks. You may not feel as ravenously hungry as you did while pregnant, and between marathon nursing sessions, dirty diapers, rocking, and just staring at your baby, you may look at the clock and realize it's noon—and you haven't had lunch or breakfast yet. But forgetting to eat is not a good way to lose the baby weight!

Here are some ways to make it easy to get enough calories and nutrition while caring for a baby:

- **Stock your fridge with healthy snacks.** Yogurt cups, cut-up cheese and vegetables, fruit, hard-boiled eggs, and pita and hummus are examples of low-fuss, low-prep foods you can easily grab and eat with one hand.
- **Set an alarm to go off every three hours.** This can help you remember that it's time to make your way to the kitchen for a little something, and will help prevent you from getting too hungry or experiencing a crash in blood sugar.
- **Keep nonperishable snacks and a bottle of water in your nursing station.** Whole-wheat crackers and peanut butter, low-sugar granola bars, and protein bars can give you a little boost when you can't get to the kitchen for something more substantial.
- **Keep taking your prenatal vitamin, or take a good multivitamin daily while breastfeeding.** Not all vitamins and supplements are created equal. If you're nursing, make sure you know that anything you're taking is safe for your baby. And if you're taking more than one supplement, add up the amounts of each nutrient you're getting to make sure you aren't getting too much. It's relatively easy to overdose on certain nutrients, like iron and vitamin A.

You need to consume an extra 200 to 500 calories a day while breastfeeding. If you lose more than 1 to 2 pounds per week, it can have a negative impact on your health and, if you're breastfeeding, can release toxins into your milk. Plus, you need adequate nutrition to keep up your energy levels. For more information on your nutritional needs in the postpartum months, see Chapter 13.

Fighting the Urge to Do Too Much

After a few weeks of being home with your baby, you may start to feel dissatisfied with the way your house is beginning to look now that the care and cleaning of your baby, not your stuff, has taken center stage. During the first week postpartum, you should remain "down" as much as you can—no housework, very little climbing stairs, and no lifting.

From week two on, you can start to slowly add little tasks back into your routine, but "slowly" is the important word here. You shouldn't be lugging baskets of laundry up and down the stairs or mopping the floors in the six weeks postpartum! Compromising your health isn't the only reason it's best not to do too much. You'll be shocked by how much and how quickly your baby changes during this time. You can always get your house clean again, but you'll never get back these early weeks with your baby.

L. Essential

Speak frankly with your husband or partner about what you need from him now that you've added a baby to the family. Many men don't respond well to hints, so give him specifics: "Honey, while I'm recovering, I can't wash the dishes or do laundry, so I'll need you to take over those tasks every day for the next six weeks."

If you have always been house proud, now is the time to relax your standards. Your visitors are coming to see you and your new baby, not your carpet and throw pillows. Ask company to help by loading the dishwasher or putting in a load of laundry during their visit. Most people are eager to help new mothers if you just tell them what you need.

If you've always been the person in your family who does all the housework, then the balance is probably going to have to shift a little—or a lot—now. The demands of caring for an infant may require you and your husband or partner to work out a more equitable way of dividing up household chores.

Rest—Even If You Don't Think You Need To

Even if you feel like you're getting plenty of sleep, you can always use more. If you're tired, it can make it much more difficult to recover well, can increase the chances that you'll develop postpartum depression, and can make it difficult for you to enjoy your baby and adjust physically and emotionally to motherhood. Even if you're feeling okay right now while skimping on sleep, you may "crash" when your baby goes through a growth spurt and wakes more at night, or when you go through a hormonal shift.

Nap when your baby naps and take every opportunity you can to rest and put your feet up, even if you can't get in a full nap. Sometimes a catnap—ten or twenty minutes of dozing—can feel wonderfully refreshing.

During the six weeks after having a baby, you'll have plenty of questions about diet, exercise, nutrition, weight loss, and getting enough sleep. In the next several chapters, we'll delve more deeply into those topics and more.

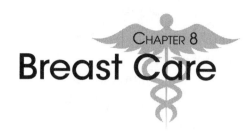

Chapter 8

Breast Care

DURING YOUR PREGNANCY, you probably noticed some changes in your breasts. You may have regarded your new breasts with delight: you'd never been so full chested before! Surprise: What's with these larger, darker nipples and bright blue veins? Or dismay: If stretch marks and sagging were part of the deal. Your breasts will continue to change throughout the postpartum period, especially in the early weeks of breastfeeding.

What's Going On in There?

When you were pregnant, your placenta told your body to start producing estrogen and progesterone, which triggered changes. Among other things, some of the fat in your breasts was replaced by glandular tissue, and as a result your breasts probably became larger and heavier—perhaps several cup sizes larger and more than a pound heavier each—and may have felt tender. Your nipples and areola, the circular pink or brown area around the nipple, probably darkened and got larger. You probably also began to see bumps on your nipples. These are called Montgomery glands, and they often become noticeable during pregnancy. They produce a substance that keeps your nipples clean and soft.

How Milk Gets Made

The hormones produced during pregnancy also stimulate the growth of milk ducts, the paths breastmilk take from the "dairy" in the alveoli, your milk-producing cells, to the milk pools under your areolas.

When your baby begins nursing after you give birth, the nerves in your breasts signal your glands to begin producing the "true" milk, which starts filling your breasts sometime between the second and fifth day postpartum.

Early Milk

Until that milk comes in, your baby will be nourished with colostrum, a sticky yellow or orange liquid that is your baby's first milk. It contains antibodies that protect your baby against disease. Colostrum will also help your baby's body eliminate meconium, the black, tar-like substance that will make up his first poops. Your breasts only produce about two tablespoons of colostrum in the first twenty-four hours after you give birth, which is just the right amount for your baby.

L. Essential

Don't worry that you aren't producing enough milk in the first few days postpartum—your baby's stomach is very small at this point, and babies are designed to pack on fat during the last few weeks of your pregnancy in anticipation of the wait for your milk's arrival.

Can You Breastfeed?

Almost all mothers are physically capable of nursing their babies. Many of the misconceptions our culture has about which mothers are able to breastfeed are based on myths and outdated information.

Small Breasts

You may worry that your small breast size will affect your body's ability to produce milk. But small breasts can produce just as much milk as larger breasts. Your breasts aren't like bottles; though they will fill up if you're late for a feeding, they'll continuously produce more milk while your baby is eating.

Large Breasts

If you have very large breasts, be sure that you have a really good-fitting, supportive nursing bra. You may have to order one through a mail-order catalog or on the Internet, as many maternity stores and department stores don't go beyond a D cup size in nursing bras. During nursing, many large-breasted women find that the football hold, over the shoulder, or lying-down position, described later in this chapter, work better than the traditional cradle hold, especially when the baby is very small. Experiment with positions to find one that's comfortable for you.

Make sure your breast is well supported throughout the feeding. You can hold your breast, or try placing a rolled-up washcloth or hand towel underneath it. When your baby is older and has better head control, you may find that you don't need as much support as in the early days. Engorgement in an already-large breast can be a challenge for a tiny-mouthed baby. You may want to express some milk first to soften the nipple. Make sure your baby's mouth is open very wide, almost like she is yawning, before you put her to the breast.

If you've had breast augmentation or breast reduction surgery, it's very possible that you'll still be able to nurse your baby, depending on the type of surgery you've had and some other factors. Talk to your doctor about your specific surgery to find out whether you'll be able to produce breastmilk. Even if you can't produce enough milk to breastfeed exclusively, you can try a supplemental nursing system, a device that allows your baby to receive formula or expressed breastmilk through a small tube that runs next to your nipple and into your baby's mouth as he nurses at your breasts. The benefits of breastfeeding go beyond just the milk, so this is a great way to have—and give to your baby—the experience of nursing even if your milk supply is low.

Nipples

Some women are afraid that the size or shape of their nipples will make nursing difficult. Inverted nipples, which point into the body rather than outside, can be an issue with early nursing but can be worked around. If you have inverted nipples, talk to a lactation consultant, La Leche League volunteer, or midwife about techniques for drawing the nipple out and making breastfeeding easier.

Breastfeeding and Lifestyle Changes

If you've gotten the idea that breastfeeding requires a Spartan diet and perfectly healthy lifestyle, you can relax a little. If you're basically healthy and well nourished and take reasonable care not to put toxic substances into your body, your milk will probably be just fine. The following are some answers to common concerns.

Diet

Most women don't have to worry about eating a special diet when they're breastfeeding. Your body will take what it needs from you to create perfect milk for your baby, and though you may have heard that certain foods can cause gas and allergies in babies, for most women this isn't a problem. Still, you'll want to be sure to eat healthy, nutritious foods—and enough of them—while breastfeeding. You'll be using an extra 200 to 500 calories per day, and you'll need to replenish your body's stores of important nutrients. As mentioned previously, many new moms find themselves forgetting to eat. Have plenty of healthy, easy-to-grab snacks on hand for nutritious on-the-go noshing.

Medication

Medications do pass from your bloodstream into your milk, though often in very small amounts. Ask your care provider or lactation consultant about the safety of over-the-counter drugs like cough syrups and antihistamines. If you're taking medication for a chronic condition, you'll want to check to see if it's safe for breastfeeding, preferably before your baby is born. If the medication isn't considered safe for nursing babies or has been shown to reduce milk supply, it's possible that your health-care provider can prescribe a breastfeeding-friendly alternative.

 ## Question

What can I take for a cold while breastfeeding?
Most prescription and over-the-counter cough syrups and cold medications are safe for use while breastfeeding. Decongestants containing pseudoephedrine have been shown to reduce milk supply in some women, so pay attention to your milk supply after taking a decongestant. If you notice a change, don't take another dose, nurse your baby, rest, and drink enough water—your supply should recover quickly.

If your doctor is not well educated about breastfeeding, he or she may recommend that you not breastfeed your baby if you're taking medication. But the many benefits of breastmilk, both for yourself and your baby, may outweigh the potential risk of a medication crossing into your milk. If it doesn't seem like your care provider is willing to work with you to make nursing your baby possible, it's a good idea to speak with a lactation consultant or find another care provider who's more supportive and knowledgeable.

Alcohol

You don't have to be a teetotaler to breastfeed. Though alcohol is completely off-limits during pregnancy, a nursing mother has a bit more freedom. Alcohol moves in and out of your milk about as quickly as it leaves your bloodstream, so a glass of wine you drink right after nursing will probably be long gone by the time your baby is hungry again. If you want to drink more than that, be aware that the alcohol will enter your milk and has the potential to make your baby dislike the taste or even cause health trouble, depending on her age, size, and how much alcohol you've had to drink. Also, some studies have linked frequent alcohol consumption with lowered milk supply and early weaning. But those party invitations on your refrigerator shouldn't keep you from breastfeeding your baby! Keep in mind that "pumping and dumping" is always an option if you'd like to indulge for a special occasion. Some moms keep a stash of pumped breast-milk in the freezer for just such an event.

 Alert

All drugs you take pass through your milk to your baby and may affect your milk supply. Street drugs in your milk can be very dangerous to your baby. Babies have died from breastmilk laced with cocaine and heroin. Drug use—including alcohol—can also keep you from being an engaged, reliable mother.

Breastfeeding Positions

When you get the hang of several different nursing positions, you can make life more convenient, help drain the breast more effectively, and avoid putting pressure on any one area of the nipple too much (which can combat nipple soreness). Some moms may also find certain positions more comfortable or easier for their babies to manage. The following are a few alternatives to the classic cradle hold.

Football Hold

This position can be more comfortable and achievable for moms with large breasts, for mothers who are recovering from a c-section, or for a premature baby. Place your baby on her side facing you, supporting her head in your hand. Instead of crossing your baby's legs in front of you as in the cradle hold, tuck her legs under your arm and put her on that side's breast, which you can support with your other hand. A pillow in your lap will help get your baby to the height of your breast and provide support.

Side-lying Position

This position allows you to get a lot of rest while nursing your baby. You and your baby will lie on your sides, facing each other. Use the crook of your arm or your forearm to support her head, and put a pillow under your head for support. Some moms rest their head on their hand, with their arm just above the baby's head. A rolled-up towel or small blanket behind your baby's back can help keep her turned toward you. Depending on the size of your breasts and your baby's head control, you may have to experiment until you find a way to make this position work for you, but the benefits to this position are worth the work!

Essential

Remember prolactin, the feel-good hormone produced when you nurse your baby? Another great "side effect" of prolactin is the fuzzy, sleepy feeling it often gives nursing moms. By getting the hang of nursing in a lying-down position, you can take advantage of these sleepy nursing sessions by getting in a little snooze while you're nursing.

Over the Shoulder

This creative position can be a lifesaver if you have very large breasts or an overactive milk-ejection reflex that has your baby gagging and choking. Since your baby will be nursing from above you, the extra milk can run out of the corners of her mouth instead of shooting down her throat.

Lie flat on your back, and put your baby over your shoulder so that her tummy is on your shoulder. She should be face-down, with her mouth coming down onto your nipple. This can be tricky to get right the first few times, so enlist help.

Leaking Milk

Leaking milk is fairly common in the first few weeks after giving birth, especially if you have a very abundant milk supply. This is a good thing. Sometimes, leaking lasts for weeks or even months after your baby is born. You may leak or spray milk during lovemaking, when you think about or hold your baby, or when you hear your baby—or another baby—crying. You may worry that you'll find yourself with a soggy shirt in public or grow tired of waking up in a wet bed.

Try these tips to reduce leaking:

- Nurse your baby frequently. If you're going to be leaving the house or making love, try nursing right beforehand to stave off leaking.
- Use flannel or cotton breast pads to catch leaks. If you use disposable breast pads, make sure they don't have a waterproof plastic layer, which can trap milk and cause yeast infections and irritation in the nipple.
- Sleep on bath towels, and wear a bra and nursing pads at night.
- If you feel tingling or the sensation of "letting down" while out in public, press your forearms firmly against your breasts. This can slow or stop the flow of milk.

Sore Nipples

One of the things moms who plan to nurse worry about the most is that it will hurt. While some soreness and tenderness is normal, there are a lot of things you can do to prevent and ease nipple pain.

Causes of Nipple Soreness

If your nipples are very sore, blistered, cracked, or bleeding, the first thing to do is make sure your baby is latching on correctly. He should be taking not just your nipple, but as much of the areola as possible, into his mouth. When he sucks, there shouldn't be any clicking sounds or dimpling in his cheeks. If he is only sucking on your nipple, not only will your nipples become very sore, but also his sucks won't stimulate your breasts to produce milk effectively. Follow the steps for good latch detailed earlier in Chapter 3. If at any time something feels or looks wrong, break the latch and try again. Some women find that expressing a little breastmilk after each feeding and rubbing it into the nipple and areola is a soothing and healing treatment. Just make sure to pat your nipple dry afterward.

Additionally, when your baby nurses in one position every time, it can create a lot of pressure on one area of your nipple or areola and can make it harder for sore, cracked nipples to heal. Try switching your baby's position each time you nurse.

Certain conditions in your baby, like nipple confusion caused by receiving bottles or pacifiers while nursing is being established, or a short frenulum (the tissue that attaches the tongue to the bottom of the mouth), also called tongue-tie, can make achieving a proper latch difficult and can exacerbate sore nipples. If you're having a hard time getting your baby to latch on or suck effectively, consult your lactation consultant, a La Leche League volunteer, or your midwife or doctor for help.

Soothe with Salve

Pure lanolin is a tried-and-true remedy for sore nipples. Its sticky, thick consistency makes it a great choice for moist wound healing: instead of allowing sores and cracks to dry and develop scabs, which are then ripped off again and again when you nurse, moist wound healing can be a more comfortable and effective way to mend nipple sores, cracks, and blisters.

Essential

For sore nipples, many women swear by an olive oil–based ointment containing comfrey, an herb that has healing qualities. Olive oil is a mild and safe base for your baby to ingest. Your health-food store may carry a healing herbal salve, or you can find one online. Just make sure all the ingredients are safe for babies.

Pure, medical-grade lanolin is readily available at drugstores and even at some grocery stores, most readily under the brand names Purelan and Lansinoh. You don't have to remove lanolin from your skin before your baby nurses. Rarely, wool allergies are linked to reactions from purified lanolin, so if you have an allergy to wool, you might want to test the lanolin on a small area of your skin first.

Alert

Though cold therapy might feel good on sore nipples, it's not a good idea to numb your nipples with ice before nursing. Serious nipple pain can be telling you that something's wrong during nursing, and by numbing it, you could allow your nipples to sustain more trauma, and the problem could get worse.

Other Remedies

Many women swear by a product called Soothies, which are cooling gel pads you apply to your breasts between feedings. The coolness can feel wonderful, and Soothies create a protective, moisturizing shield between your nipple and bra or shirt. Another option is a breast shell (not to be confused with a breast shield, which can cause supply issues and should only be used under the recommendation of an experienced lactation consultant, or your midwife or doctor). Breast shells are worn between feedings and help keep your nipple from sticking to your bra or shirt, which can be painful and reopen sores. They are also sometimes used to draw out inverted nipples.

Keep Nursing

When your nipples hurt, it can be hard to even think about nursing without cringing. But as hard as it can be, putting off feedings out of fear often makes matters worse; if your breasts become engorged, nursing will hurt even worse and you may develop an infection. Nursing more often, not less often, is the best plan of attack for sore nipples.

Try nursing on the least-sore side first. Once milk gets flowing, your baby may not suck as hard on the sore side. If your breasts are very engorged and it's making it difficult for your baby to nurse, try pumping or hand expressing a little milk to soften the nipple and ease latch-on. If you're really desperate, try pumping at every other feeding, or pumping at the beginning of a feeding, to soften the nipple and make it easier for your baby to latch on.

Ruling Out Thrush

Very sore nipples can sometimes be caused by thrush, an overabundance of yeast that can manifest on your nipples or in your baby's mouth. Thrush can be easy to miss and can make nursing very painful, so it's always a good idea to rule it out if you're experiencing persistent or severe nipple soreness. If you have a thrush infection, your nipples may look shiny, puffy, pink, blistered, or flaky. Your baby's mouth may have small white spots in it, and he may cry and pull away when he nurses. Sometimes, though, thrush doesn't show any symptoms in a baby, and the only symptom you experience could be pain.

⌐ Essential

The pain of thrush is often described as burning, stabbing, or sharp, and may radiate through the milk ducts and even into your armpit. Generally, the pain is worst during latch-on but persists throughout the feeding. Garden-variety tender nipples usually get better by the end of the first week or so, but thrush tends to get worse, not better, with time.

If your water was broken or leaking for more than twenty-four hours before you went into labor, if you tested positive for group B strep bacteria late in your pregnancy, or if you experienced any symptoms of infection after your baby was born, there's a good chance you received antibiotic treatment, which can also increase your chances of developing thrush. Or, if your baby was given antibiotics, he could have developed thrush and then passed it back to you.

If you think you might have thrush, don't hesitate to start treatment. Once the "yeastie beasties" have a foothold, they usually won't go away without a nudge—and without treatment, the pain will just get worse. Or, the infection might spread to your baby, making it more difficult to nip the problem in the bud.

Prevention

Yeast grows best in warm, moist environments, so make sure you keep your nipples dry between feedings. Pat your nipples dry or expose them to the air after each feeding, and change your nursing pads or nursing bra often. Wash bras and reusable nursing pads daily in hot water, and dry them completely before putting them back on. If your nipples become cracked or blistered because of poor latch or other issues, it can create an environment that yeast can thrive in. Keep your nipples dry (when not in use) and moisturized.

Treatment

Your health-care provider can prescribe you an antifungal medication, like Diflucan or Nystatin. It can be difficult to diagnose nipple thrush, and women often have a hard time getting their doctor to prescribe the medication. Also, the drugs can be really expensive, especially if you don't have prescriptive insurance. If you can't get your doctor to prescribe you an antifungal, or if you're prescribed one that doesn't work, don't worry—you still have several treatment options.

Over-the-counter Antifungal Creams

Creams containing the active ingredient miconazole or clotrimazole can be used directly on your nipples after each feeding. Dr. Jack Newman, an internationally recognized breastfeeding expert, recommends asking your pharmacist to make up this "all-purpose nipple ointment" for the treatment of thrush and other causes of sore nipples:

- 15 grams 2 percent mupirocin ointment (not cream)
- 15 grams 0.1 percent betamethasone ointment (not cream)

If this is unavailable, mometasone ointment can be substituted. Don't mix ointments and creams together.

Add miconazole powder, so that the final concentration is 2 percent miconazole. If miconazole is unavailable, clotrimazole powder can be substituted. Apply this combination sparingly after each feeding, but not at the same time as gentian violet. Do not wash or wipe it off; according to Dr. Newman, this formula is safe for your baby to ingest.

Gentian Violet

You can still find this inexpensive, old-time remedy in many drugstores, but you might have to ask the pharmacist for help. Gentian violet is a dye with powerful antifungal properties and is sold in powder and liquid form. Dilute the gentian violet until you have a 0.25 to 0.5 percent solution, and apply it to your breasts once a day with a cotton swab before nursing your baby. That way, his mouth will get treated too (don't worry, a small amount of gentian violet is safe for your baby to swallow).

Treatment with gentian violet can be extremely messy, and gentian violet will stain your clothing and temporarily turn your baby's lips and mouth purple. To make cleanup easier, try rubbing a little olive oil on and around your baby's lips and cheeks before a feeding. The oil will provide a barrier between your baby's skin and the dye, and may reduce staining.

While health-care providers around the world recommend gentian violet regularly as a safe, effective treatment for thrush, some experts aren't convinced it's completely safe. Gentian violet should be a short-term, infrequent treatment. If your symptoms aren't better after treating with gentian violet for a few days, or if your thrush continues to recur, talk to your health-care provider about other options.

Acidopholus

Yeast and other microorganisms are always present in a healthy body, but usually, they keep one another in check. When "good" bacteria are wiped out of your system, the yeast can grow unchecked. Restoring the levels of healthy bacteria in your body is your first line of defense against thrush infections. Plus, regularly consuming lactobacillus acidopholus is good for your digestive system. As mentioned previously, you can take acidopholus in pill form or get it in yogurt containing live cultures. It works topically, too: open an acidopholus capsule or take a little plain yogurt and swab it on your nipples.

Other Breast Issues

Unfortunately, sore nipples and thrush aren't the only breast problems you might experience during your first few weeks postpartum. Engorgement and clogged ducts are also possibilities, but the good news is that a few simple methods can alleviate both problems fairly quickly.

Engorgement

When your milk comes in, you may experience swollen, engorged breasts. This is due not only to the milk filling your breasts, but also to increased blood flow to the area. Engorgement can be quite painful. Your engorged breasts may grow several cup sizes very quickly and feel warm and hard. It's a good idea to wear a supportive bra with enough room for your larger breasts. A halter top that supports from below without pressure may be a great solution.

Nursing often in the first few days is a good way to keep the milk moving and prevent breasts from becoming too engorged. Also, massaging your breasts in a warm shower or bath can feel good and can help move some of the milk out of the ducts.

Essential

Cold therapy is soothing on engorged breasts and can help decrease swelling. You can also try a refrigerated rice sock (see Chapter 1 for directions), an ice pack, a zipper-lock bag full of ice cubes, or a bag of frozen vegetables wrapped in a washcloth.

If your breasts are very engorged, cabbage leaves can make a soothing treatment. Buy a cabbage, peel and clean the leaves, and store them in the refrigerator. Get enough leaves to completely cover your breasts, all the way from one side to the other, and right up to the area under your armpit. Break the cabbage's "veins" by gently crushing them, and then tuck the leaves into your bra or lie on your back and relax with the leaves resting on your breasts. The leaves will be cool and soothing; you should start to feel some relief within a few hours. Replace the leaves whenever they look wilted, or every two hours. Only use cabbage leaves while you're engorged—if you use them too long, they can decrease your milk supply.

Bottle Feeding and Engorgement

If you won't be nursing, you will have to take measures to prevent engorgement in the first few days. Wear a snug-fitting bra, or wrap your breasts with stretchy bandages. Cabbage leaves and cold therapy, as described earlier in this chapter, may help with discomfort and relieve engorgement. You'll want to remove some milk from the breasts, but not enough to stimulate milk production—pumping just a little every four to five hours or hand expressing milk in the shower may do the trick.

Clogged Ducts

Clogged ducts can happen when milk isn't moved out of the breasts often enough. If your breast is compressed by an underwire bra, by tight clothing, or by sleeping on your chest, you can also develop clogged ducts. If you can feel a hard spot in your breast, if there's localized soreness below the skin, or if your breast has an area that's red or warm to the touch, it could indicate a clogged duct.

Try massaging your breast from the armpit out toward the nipple to break up the clog and move it out. A little olive oil helps your hands to move smoothly over your tender breast without too much pressure. This can be more effective when done in a warm shower or bath, or after applying a warm, wet washcloth or heated rice sock to the breast for a few minutes. Some women find relief from clogged ducts by hovering on all fours over their baby and massaging the affected breast while nursing. This may feel silly (like you have udders instead of breasts), but letting your breast hang free can remove the compression that can sometimes slow the milk flow and cause or worsen clogs.

Everyday Breast Care

When you've gotten past the first few weeks postpartum and nursing is going well, you won't need to do much to care for your breasts. Rinsing them with water in the shower is sufficient—don't wash your nipples with soap, as that can be drying and irritating to the nipple's tissue. If you're not nursing, you may leak a little milk for weeks or even months after giving birth even if you never breastfeed.

If you've gotten off to a rough start with breastfeeding, don't worry—sore nipples and the oversupply and undersupply issues that sometimes make the first weeks of nursing difficult almost always work themselves out after a few weeks. As your body begins to recognize your baby's feeding patterns, it will adjust the output of milk to meet your baby's needs without oversupply. Your breasts will soften, your nipples will toughen up, and you'll get the hang of recognizing your baby's hunger signals and getting him onto your breast. It is truly all worth it for the benefits to both of you.

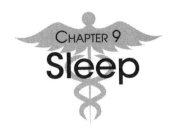

CHAPTER 9

Sleep

THE IMPORTANCE OF A GOOD night's sleep should not be underestimated! Studies have shown that sleep deprivation can lead to lowered alertness and productivity. Lack of sleep can make it difficult to be an engaged, happy mother, and a lack of quality sleep has been linked to postpartum depression. It's not always easy to get enough sleep while your baby is very young, but there are ways you can get the most from your sleeping time without weaning or "training" your newborn.

How Much Newborn Babies Sleep

Every new mom gets this question at least a dozen times from well-meaning friends and relatives in the early months postpartum: "Does your baby sleep through the night yet?"

This phrase can be misleading. According to experts, "sleeping through the night" is defined by a baby sleeping six hours at a stretch. That means if you put your baby to bed at 8 P.M., and he wakes up at 2 A.M., technically, he's slept through the night. Keep that in mind when you hear or read experts say that your baby should sleep through the night by three or four months of age. Sure, technically your baby's sleep might be meeting the "through the night" criteria, but it sure won't feel like it to you!

Why He Wakes Up

A baby's stomach is very small, and doesn't hold enough milk to keep him satisfied for long. In fact, if you have a premature or very sleepy baby, you may actually have to wake him up every three to four hours to eat. It can be dangerous for small babies to routinely go longer between feedings. Newborns don't understand that night is for sleeping, and that day is for playing and eating. They only know that it's been a few hours since they last ate, and they're hungry.

The good news is that newborn babies do sleep a lot: up to sixteen hours a day, just not all at once. Biologically, a young infant is programmed to wake up and eat, sometimes as often as every two hours (or sometimes even more often). This is normal and natural, and not a sign that your baby is "spoiled" or "a bad sleeper."

Baby's the Boss

In these early months, trying to control your baby's feeding or sleeping habits is an exercise in futility: it probably won't work, and if it does, it will cause you and your baby plenty of grief along the way. Leaving a baby to "cry it out" at this young age is not only cruel to the baby, who is hungry and doesn't understand why nobody is feeding him, but is also heart-wrenching for mothers.

L. Essential

Keeping your baby awake when he's tired during the day in the hopes that he'll sleep better at night may backfire: babies need to nap, and research shows that an overtired baby might have an even more difficult time winding down at the end of the day.

As your baby grows, he'll start to go longer between feedings, increase his time spent sleeping at a stretch, and become more receptive to you directing his sleeping and eating habits.

You Need Your Sleep, Too

Many new moms don't notice the effects of sleep deprivation right away. But after a while, the debt you incur from missing out on sleep begins to add up, until it begins to affect your productivity, alertness, and even your moods. Your memory can become less sharp; you can be more prone to accidents or injuries; and your may feel irritable, sad, or depressed.

Even if you aren't significantly sleep deprived, it can be frustrating to go from the relative luxury of a full, straight night's sleep at night to waking every two hours or so. Often, mothers begin to worry that their babies aren't sleeping enough or that they aren't putting them to bed correctly, which just causes more anxiety and stress. It helps to have a realistic idea of how much you can expect your newborn to sleep in any one stretch.

With a baby that wakes every couple of hours to eat, how can you avoid dangerous and debilitating sleep deprivation? You probably won't be able to count on eight hours of uninterrupted sleep at night for the foreseeable future, so you'll have to get creative.

Flexible Routines Can Help

Instead of trying to stick to a strict schedule, try establishing a flexible routine. If you follow the same basic pattern every day—for instance, dinner, then reading, then a bath, then bedtime—your baby will soon begin to associate bedtime with sleep. It can also help you feel sleepy at around the same time every day, which can be helpful if you have trouble falling asleep due to anxiety or restlessness.

Sleep When Your Baby Sleeps

Staying up late watching Letterman may be a thing of the past, unless your baby is a night owl. When you've got a newborn, your opportunity for nighttime sleep is limited, and it makes sense to take advantage of every second. Later, when he's sleeping longer at a stretch and his routine starts to even out, you can plan for some "you" time after he goes to bed at night. But for the time being, unless your baby is a spectacular snoozer, you'll probably be better off turning in when he does.

When the Sandman Doesn't Come

Even if you're exhausted, you may have trouble going to sleep on command, especially if your baby falls asleep a lot earlier than your usual bedtime or you're feeling anxious. Here are some tips for helping you relax and catch some z's:

- If you're too anxious to sleep, try a meditation, visualization, or hypnosis CD. These can help you turn off the chatter in your brain and relax enough to fall asleep.
- If your mind is racing and full of thoughts, try getting those thoughts out on paper right before bed. Writing in a journal can be a great way to clear your mind and ready yourself for a good night's sleep.
- Make sure your room isn't too hot or too cold, and that it's dark and quiet enough.
- Watching TV right before bed may make it more difficult for you to go to sleep, particularly if you watch a disturbing, scary, or exciting program.
- Avoid caffeine. This includes chocolate, coffee, and many kinds of teas and sodas.
- If you absolutely can't sleep, it may be better to get out of bed or read for a while than to lie there tossing and turning.
- That old standby, warm milk, can really help put you to sleep. Try adding some honey or brown sugar and vanilla for a tasty way to wind down before bed.
- Take a warm bath with your baby, tuck yourselves into bed, and nurse yourselves to sleep.

Mastering Naps

Your baby might not be sleeping through the night—or anything close to it—yet, but chances are good he takes plenty of naps. You can take advantage of his sleepy time by getting a little shuteye yourself.

According to the National Sleep Foundation, there are three types of naps: planned napping, when you take a nap before you actually get sleepy because you know you'll be missing out on sleep later; emergency napping, which happens when you are suddenly very tired and feel like you need to go to sleep; and habitual napping, which is when you take a nap at the same time each day. As a new mom, you might be employing all three of these types of naps—sometimes, more than one in the same day.

Make Napping Easy

Some people have a hard time falling asleep in the middle of the day, even if they are sleep deprived. Make sure the environment you've set up is conducive to sleep. The room shouldn't be too hot, too cold, or too bright. Draw the curtains or close the blinds. And make sure you won't be interrupted by unwanted noises. For example, turn the ringer off on your phone.

Essential

If background noises disturb you, try running a fan or humidifier to create a low hum. There are even machines that play sounds of ocean waves or other white noise, which may keep you from focusing on the bothersome sound and help lull you—and your baby—to sleep.

If you have mastered the lying-down position while breastfeeding, outlined in Chapter 8, you're ahead of the game—the hormones released while nursing your baby can relax you and make you sleepy, and the two of you can drift off together. Even if your baby doesn't take a long nap after he nurses, you might be able to get in a good twenty minutes or so while he's eating, which will at least leave you more refreshed and alert for the short term.

Take What You Can Get

You may notice that you're groggy and disoriented after taking a long nap. Naps that last longer than twenty or thirty minutes aren't usually recommended as part of a regular sleep routine, since they can leave you feeling worse on waking and also interfere with falling asleep at the proper time at night. But while you have an infant, you can't count on falling asleep at the same time every night, and you may need all the extra slumber you can get. If you approach sleep with a grab-it-while-you-can attitude in these early days, you will be in a much better frame of mind for developing sleep routines later, when your baby is ready for it.

Even if you can't fall asleep, just lying down with your baby and resting as much as possible is vital during the first weeks postpartum. You need to rest to recover as quickly and fully as possible, and putting your feet up and closing your eyes whenever your baby is napping is a nice way to work breaks into your day and help you fight the temptation to be too busy.

Where Should Your Baby Sleep?

In many cultures, co-sleeping is, and always has been, the norm. If you think about it, the practice of mothers and babies sleeping together makes a lot of sense: babies are comforted by the closeness of their mothers and often sleep better, and mothers will be comforted by knowing their baby is okay and may also sleep better. Plus, nothing is as easy and restful for a nursing mom as simply lifting her top, latching the baby on, and dozing off again.

In the United States, however, co-sleeping isn't considered the norm. Our culture relies on bassinettes, cribs, and other baby beds, and often encourages independence right from the start. You may even have heard that co-sleeping is dangerous and increases the risk of sudden infant death syndrome (SIDS). But many experts agree that there is a safe way to practice co-sleeping, just as there are safe and unsafe ways to use cribs and other baby beds. There are many benefits to co-sleeping: it's easy and convenient for nursing mothers, and may help you sleep better if you don't have to get out of bed every time your baby wants to eat.

Essential

Some studies suggest that co-sleeping may actually reduce the risk of SIDS. Deep, unbroken sleep seems to make it more likely that babies will get into trouble with breathing, and when babies sleep close to their mothers, they sleep more lightly and breathe more evenly.

Co-sleeping is not an all-or-nothing proposition. Many mothers start their babies out in a crib, then bring them to their own bed to sleep from the first feeding on. Other parents sleep with their babies during special circumstances. If you decide to co-sleep, you may receive criticism from family and friends, but you may also be pleasantly surprised to find out just how many parents sleep with their children at least some of the time. Do you know anyone who has never taken a nap alongside their baby?

Sleep Safely

If you plan to bring your baby into your bed some or all of the time, please follow these safety guidelines:

- Your mattress should be flat and firm, and there should be no crevices or gaps between the mattress and the wall or headboard that your baby can slip into. To keep your baby from rolling off the bed, simply put your mattress on the floor, or use a mesh guardrail. Make sure the guardrail is intended to be used by babies. Do not put your baby to sleep on a waterbed, sofa, pillow-top mattress, or any other surface that could trap his head or create pockets of air for him to breathe again and again.

- Make sure your bottom sheet is securely tucked under the mattress edges and won't be pulled loose during the night. A fitted sheet's elastic could wrap over your baby's head.
- Be sure your mattress is big enough to accommodate you, your husband or partner, and a baby comfortably. Many families look at this as a good opportunity to upgrade to a king-sized bed.
- Check your mattress every night to be sure the fitted sheets are still secure and that there is no space between the wall or headboard and the mattress.
- Your baby should sleep between you and the wall or guardrail. Mothers have an instinctual awareness of where their baby is at night, but fathers and other family members may not have the same ability.
- Don't ever sleep with your baby if you've been drinking or if you are using any medication that might make you sleepy.
- Make sure there are no pillows, blankets, or other items in the bed that could cover your baby's head.
- Don't dress your baby too warmly or cover him up with heavy blankets.

Question

I'm overweight. Can I sleep with my baby?
Evidence shows that babies are at a higher risk when they co-sleep with obese mothers. The danger is that the sleeping mother's weight will create a dip in the mattress that a baby could roll into. If you are very heavy, a sidecar arrangement, described on the next page, may be a better choice.

But Won't I Roll Over on Him?

Many mothers express fear that they'll roll over on or suffocate their babies at night. But research has shown that this is very seldom a real danger, unless the mother is under the influence of medication, alcohol, or other drugs, or is obese. Most co-sleeping mothers report that they wake up long before their baby gets hungry, detecting small movements, sighs, or even the smacking of tiny lips in their sleep. New moms are hardwired not to sleep heavily or soundly—they're on the alert in case their baby needs them.

 Alert

> Safe co-sleeping is dependent on a mother being aware, even in her sleep, of all her baby's sounds and motions. If you aren't wakened by your baby's slight movement or soft sounds, you may want to consider using a sidecar arrangement instead.

Try a Sidecar

If you don't feel comfortable having your baby in your bed, consider a sidecar arrangement. You can purchase a special "co-sleeper," a small bed that butts up against your own bed and provides a firm, safe place for your infant to sleep. Another option is placing a crib alongside your bed and adjusting the crib mattress to be the same height as your mattress, with the guardrail down. This option will take up more room, but will be useful much longer than a co-sleeper, which your baby will soon outgrow.

Using the sidecar arrangement, you can pull your baby close to you while he's nursing, and then gently slide him back over to the co-sleeper when he's done. Even if your baby doesn't end back up in the sidecar every night, it can act as an extension of your sleeping space, making the bed feel roomier. That way, everybody can spread out a bit, and you'll be reassured that if your baby rolls, he won't fall off the bed.

Other Arrangements

The next best choice is having your baby in a bassinette or cradle near your bed at night. This arrangement is recommended by the American Academy of Pediatrics because it facilitates breastfeeding and keeps you and your baby close by one another. That way, she'll have the benefit of smelling you close by and hearing your breathing, you'll be less anxious about whether she's doing okay, and you will probably hear her waking up in time to feed her before she gets really hungry and upset.

If your baby sleeps in her own room, use a baby monitor to hear her stirring before she wakes up completely. Once a baby is upset enough that you could hear her crying down the hall, you will both have a much harder time going back to sleep.

Maximizing Sleep Time

When your baby wakes at night, change her diaper first if she needs it. Keep the lights low and be quiet as you change her.

It's easy to keep diaper changes low-key if you're co-sleeping or using a sidecar. You can keep diapers and other changing gear on your bedside table and simply change your baby right on your bed to avoid waking her more. Once your baby is clean and dry, you can get comfortable and nurse her back to sleep. Don't worry too much about the "danger" of your baby getting used to falling asleep at the breast in these early weeks. The goal here is sleep for your baby, and sleep for you. There are a lot of techniques for helping babies learn to sleep on their own, but they will require energy from you, and you'll probably have to sacrifice some sleep yourself to make them work. As your baby matures and you're both settling into a routine, you can begin helping her fall asleep on her own by nursing her until she's very sleepy, then removing the breast from her mouth and allowing her to fall asleep without it. But in these early weeks, don't worry about "training" your baby—just get as much sleep as you can.

Ĺ Essential

You may have heard that giving your breastfed baby formula or rice cereal in a bottle will help her sleep better. These "tricks" don't work and may make matters worse—the formula could upset her tummy, and rice cereal is not safe for newborn babies to eat or drink. They may keep your baby asleep longer, but that's only because they are poorly digested and sit in her stomach, making her feel full.

If, despite taking measures to make sure you're sleeping as much as possible, you find that you're exhausted all the time, you must ask for help. Sleep deprivation can make you an unsafe driver and a less-attentive mother, and it can limit your ability to enjoy and bond with your baby. Tell your husband or partner you need him and let him know specifically how he can help you get enough sleep.

Just remember one thing: Having your partner feed your baby formula or pumped milk may look like an attractive option, but this can have drawbacks. You will probably wake up anyway, uncomfortably full of milk, and you'll risk either developing clogged ducts or mastitis or experience a drop in milk supply.

Luckily, nursing mothers can get nighttime help from Dad without weaning or giving bottles. Here are some breastfeeding-friendly ways to let your partner take over some of the night shift:

- Dad can handle the nighttime routine a few days a week while you go to bed early. You'll get in a few hours of sleep before your baby goes down for the night.
- Some mornings, your husband or partner can get up with the baby in the morning and let you sleep in.

- If your baby sleeps in his own bed or in another room, your partner can take over everything but the feeding. Dad can go get him when he wakes up, change his diaper, bring him to you for a feeding, and then settle him back down into his bed when he's done. Meanwhile you can doze through the feeding and never leave the comfort of your bed, with the assurance that your baby will be cared for while you sleep.

If both you and your partner are exhausted or you're a single mom, it's time to call in the help of family, friends, or a postpartum doula to help you. See if a friend can come over and care for your baby for a few hours while you sleep. So what if it is the middle of the afternoon? When you're really sleep deprived, any shuteye feels amazing and will help refill your sleep account.

 Alert

If you ever feel so tired you can't stay awake, you think you might hurt your baby, or you feel desperate or suicidal, it is an emergency situation and you must do what you can to get some rest. Call your partner, a trusted friend, or your care provider immediately.

Ignore the Critics

Despite what experts and the self-proclaimed experts in your family say, there's no one right way for a baby to sleep. Listen to your baby and yourself; if where or when your baby is sleeping doesn't seem to be working or you are simply not getting enough sleep to function well, consider making a change. But if you're happy and rested and your baby is thriving, there's no reason to cut out nighttime nursing, put your baby on a strict sleeping or feeding schedule, or move her to another room.

You can always change your sleeping arrangement later if it stops working for you or your baby. There's only a problem if somebody in the family is not getting the rest he or she needs. Otherwise, you can ignore your critics and feel good about the choices you've made for your family.

Essential

Breastfeeding is not just about nutrition. Your baby may wake to nurse for a variety of reasons: she may be hungry, she may be uncomfortable, or she may simply crave nurturing from you. And you may find that you enjoy the quiet time with her in the middle of the night.

It can be hard to imagine when you're bleary eyed and exhausted, walking the floor with a crying baby at 3 A.M., but things will begin to get better. If your baby is very fussy or colicky, you can expect it to get better around the time he's three months old. As his digestive system matures, he'll be able to go longer and longer between feedings, and he'll sleep longer and longer at night. Believe it or not, you will sleep again.

Skin and Hair Care

DURING PREGNANCY, YOUR SKIN and hair may have gone through many changes: your hair may have become fuller or frizzier, and your skin might have developed darker spots or a variety of lumps and bumps. After your baby is born, many of those changes will fade away, only to be replaced by new changes as your hormone levels fluctuate and finally even out. Often, you can deal with these changes by mixing up your beauty routine or selecting new products for your new skin and hair.

Skin Changes Left Over from Pregnancy

If you became hairier, blotchy, bumpy, or itchy during pregnancy, you're probably looking forward to your skin getting back to normal. Eventually it will, but it could take some time and further changes before everything settles down. The following sections cover some common pregnancy-related skin issues, and what you can expect now that you're no longer pregnant.

Skin Tags

These small, fleshy lumps of skin are common in pregnant women and can develop anywhere, but are most common in the areas where you have folds, like your armpits or the crease of your thighs. Once here, a skin tag usually won't budge on its own, but it can easily be removed in a doctor's office.

Question

> **Can I get rid of skin tags at home?**
> There are several popular home remedies for skin tags. You can try painting over the tag with clear nail polish or tying a piece of dental floss tightly around the base of the tag. Both these methods can kill the skin tag, which will fall off.

Dark Patches

If you developed dark splotches or other changes to the pigmentation of your skin while you were pregnant—called cholasma, melasma, or the mask of pregnancy, they'll go away when your hormone levels go back to their normal, nonpregnant state, generally within a few months of birth. Any other changes to your skin's pigment, such as the *linea nigra*, the dark line that may have developed down your belly, or darker freckles or birthmarks, will also fade.

Certain things can make these pigment changes remain longer or even come back, such as exposure to the sun, or use of hormonal contraceptives containing estrogen, like birth-control pills, the patch, or the ring. You can switch to a nonhormonal or progestin-only method of birth control, which is a better choice if you're breastfeeding, anyway. If the dark spots on your skin don't fade, a dermatologist may be able to lighten them with a bleaching cream, chemical peel, or other type of medication.

Excess Face and Body Hair

During pregnancy, you might have noticed certain parts of your body becoming fuzzier than they were before. Excess hair on your face, neck, legs, and pubic area should decrease after your baby is born, but some women notice that they keep a little extra hair in certain areas after giving birth.

Itching, Rashes, and Bumps

When you were pregnant, you may have suffered from hormone-induced itching, bumps, or rashes. One common and very uncomfortable culprit is pruritic urticarial papules and plaques of pregnancy (PUPPPs), an extremely itchy condition that generally clears up after pregnancy. It doesn't always go away immediately after giving birth, but should clear up as soon as the hormone levels causing the rash even out.

 Alert

> If you develop a rash, hives, or itching while taking a medication, such as an antibiotic for a postpartum infection, tell your care provider immediately. Itching and rashes are common symptoms of allergic reactions to medication, which can be serious.

Itching, hives, and rashes can also be caused by different allergic reactions and sensitivities. Are you using a new detergent for your baby's clothing, or a lotion with ingredients you might be reacting to? If you're having trouble sleeping or can't stop scratching, talk to your doctor or midwife, who may prescribe a topical steroid, antihistamine, or alternative.

Excessive Sweating

During pregnancy, your body's fluid volume increased by 50 percent. If you had an epidural or IV during labor and delivery, even more fluids were pushed into your system. Then, after your baby was born, your body wanted to gradually get rid of all those extra fluids. For you, this may mean increased sweating, especially at night. The sweating can seem excessive—you may wake up in soaking-wet sheets—but it is normal and will usually decrease by the end of the first week postpartum, though it may not go away entirely for a month or more. Hormonal fluctuations can also contribute to increased sweating. Try wearing all-cotton clothing at night and sleeping with a towel under your body. One hundred percent cotton sheets and mattress pads may also help make your bed a more comfortable place to sweat it out. Ask your husband or partner to strip and wash your sheets daily so that you go to bed in a comfortable, clean place every night.

Persistent sweating, very dry skin, rashes, and excessive hair loss can all be caused by thyroid dysfunction, a condition marked by an over- or under-functioning thyroid. Thyroid dysfunction afflicts up to 10 percent of postpartum women. Other symptoms of postpartum thyroiditis may include extreme fatigue, anxiety, or irritability, and excessive weight loss or the inability to lose weight. Talk to your doctor or midwife if you have these symptoms.

Stretch Marks

Stretch marks are a very common side effect of the often-rapid growth and weight gain you probably experienced during pregnancy. On some women, stretch marks can look very severe—they may be raw, painful, or even bleed, and can be found anywhere you may have gained weight or grown quickly—breasts, abdomen, hips, thighs, and even arms. Though the idea that stretch marks can be prevented by moisturizing the skin seems to persist, a large part of what causes stretch marks has to do with your genetic predisposition to the marks, as well as your diet, and how much you grew, and how fast, while pregnant.

Now that the stretch marks are here, you've got some possibilities for treatment. Dermabrasion, chemical peels, and laser treatments have been touted as ways to help your stretch marks blend in with the rest of your skin, and some treatments are said to help the skin regain some of its elasticity. Speak to a dermatologist or cosmetic surgeon if you're really unhappy with how your skin looks after a year or so. He or she will be able to suggest the best treatment method for you.

Alert

> Some medications, such as Retin A, have been shown to be effective at fading stretch marks when used soon after you give birth. But not all of them are safe for breastfeeding, and may carry a risk of birth defects if you were to get pregnant again during treatment.

Keep in mind that no treatment is likely to completely eradicate the marks pregnancy left on your body, and if you have more children, the stretch marks will probably reappear. It's probably a better idea to wait until some time has passed after the birth of your last baby before you make any permanent cosmetic changes. That way, you'll see what your true "new" body looks like and will have time to become more comfortable with it before you spend the time and expense on cosmetic treatment.

In the meantime, your stretch marks will eventually fade and lighten, from purply red to a silvery white. Your skin will probably also tighten up a bit, which can make your stretch marks look less prominent. After they have a chance to get used to them, many women proudly carry their stretch marks as a sign of the changes their bodies went through during pregnancy on their journey to motherhood.

Changes to Your Complexion

Just as pregnancy may have caused your skin to flip-flop from oily to dry or vice versa, the hormonal changes you'll go through after birth, and the stress and fatigue of having a new baby can bring with them major changes to your complexion. If you had clear skin before, you may notice pimples now; or if you had oilier skin, it may be very dry now. You also might find that you're not keeping up with your previous face-care regimen, which could lead to breakouts or dryness. Here are a few tips for working skin care into your routine, whether your skin is dry, oily, or a little of both.

Dry Skin

If your skin feels tight, itchy, or rough, or if it looks flaky, you've probably got dry skin. You'll want to use a creamy cleanser that doesn't foam up—look for one specially formulated for dry skin. Avoid using soap, which can be drying, and don't put your face directly into hot water—which means no standing with your face pointed into the shower stream. Exfoliate once a week, and be sure to moisturize. You may need to use a heavier, creamier moisturizer than the one you used to use.

▌, Essential

Oatmeal makes a soothing natural remedy for itching, rashy skin. You can purchase oatmeal treatments at your pharmacy or health-food store, or try this: put a cup or two of dry oatmeal into a clean knee-high stocking, tie the end closed, and drop it into a warm bath.

It's not just your face that may suffer from dry skin. The drop in your body's production of estrogen after you give birth may leave the rest of your body feeling dry, itchy, and rough, too.

Avoid taking a shower in very hot water or lounging in a hot bathtub, since the hot water can further sap moisture from your skin. Exfoliate in a warm shower—a washcloth will do, but a nice-smelling moisturizing scrub may feel more luxurious—and follow immediately with a layer of thick lotion while your skin is still damp. Lotions containing aloe and shea butter can be very moisturizing. Also, you might want to consider a lotion that contains alpha-hydroxy acids, which can help your body shed dead, flaky skin cells. These products can be irritating to sensitive skin, so try a little on your inner elbow before you put it all over your body.

Oily Skin

If you're able to soak up oil onto a tissue or blotting paper about twenty minutes after washing your face, you probably have oily skin. A cleanser that foams or suds up during washing is the best way to wash away excess oil. Exfoliate several times a week with a gentle scrub or washcloth, but don't use an exfoliant that's too rough, because it may actually stimulate your glands to create more oil. A light, oil-free moisturizer that doesn't clog pores will help your skin stay soft without adding more grease. There are also products that moisturize your skin while helping the surface stay matte and keeping oil at bay.

 Alert

Be careful if you use bath oil or an oily exfoliating product, like the popular sugar and salt scrubs sold in bath and body stores. These can make your bathtub or shower extremely slippery for several showers, making it a potentially dangerous place for both you and your baby.

Combination Skin

If your cheeks feel tight but your nose and chin are oily, you may have what's known as combination skin. This can be a little trickier to care for, since you won't want to do the same thing to your nose as you do to your cheeks. Use a gentle cleanser made for combination skin all over, and then concentrate your moisturizer just on your cheeks and other dry areas. If you rely on your moisturizer's SPF factor to shield your skin from the sun, you may want to switch to an oil-free sunscreen for all-over protection and then follow with a thicker moisturizer on your dry spots.

Acne

Acne is very common in the first couple of months after giving birth, and you may be dismayed to see that it isn't limited to your face—your back, shoulders, and even your rear end may be affected by breakouts. This is due to postpartum hormone fluctuations and should clear up soon. In the meantime, do the best you can to keep your skin clean.

 Fact

Over-the-counter acne medications containing benzoyl peroxide or salicyclic acid are compatible with breastfeeding, and some topical medications that require a prescription, like Differin and MetroGel, are also considered safe by breastfeeding experts.

If you decide to see a dermatologist for acne treatment while breastfeeding, make sure your doctor knows you're nursing and check to be sure that any medication you're prescribed is safe for your baby. Keep in mind that oral antibiotics can lead to yeast infections and nipple thrush, so they should be a last resort.

Making Time for a Skin-care Routine

If you're falling into bed exhausted every night and waking up on the go every morning, remembering your facial-care routine might seem out of the question. But if cranky skin is getting you down, it's probably worth setting aside a few minutes each day to cleanse and moisturize. Here are a few tips to guide you:

- **Make it part of your routine.** Now that your time is no longer wholly your own, you may find that you rely more and more on routines to help you get important things done. Caring for your skin should be a part of that routine. For example, you can wash and moisturize your face while waiting for your tea to brew every morning.

- **Find new products that fit your new skin.** If you usually wear makeup, you may need to experiment with different formulations or brands to find a good match for your skin. It's more expensive than buying your makeup from the drugstore, but it might be worthwhile to seek out a department store where the salespeople can recommend products for your skin type and give you an in-store demonstration before you buy.
- **Make it easy on yourself.** Choose products that are easy to use, multifunctional, and require little fuss or time. Even the type of bottle (does it require two hands to open?) may make the difference between a product you'll be able to use easily while holding your baby or one you'll be more likely to skip.
- **Keep it clean.** Heavy makeup isn't just time-consuming to apply, but also it clogs pores and takes a lot longer to wash away completely. Who needs it, especially if you'll be spending a lot of time at home?

Changes to Your Hair

You probably noticed some changes to your hair while you were pregnant. During pregnancy, your hair is in a growth phase, meaning it doesn't shed in the same volume as nonpregnant hair does. For some women this means lustrous, glossy, thick locks; for others, it's a recipe for a bushy 'do with a life of its own. Whatever pregnancy did to your hair, during the postpartum months you can expect some more changes as your hormones once again fluctuate. A drop in estrogen production equals dryness for many women, and that can be reflected in your hair's texture. Or, you may notice that once normal or dry hair is on the oily side now.

Before you reach for your usual bottle of shampoo and conditioner on your next shopping trip, or put your hair in the same old 'do, take a close look at your hair. Might a new formula or style be a better choice for you? Whether your hair is thin or coarse, here are some product and styling tips that might work well for you.

Fact

> Many women report that their hair not only thins out after pregnancy but also changes texture—from curly to straight or wavy to curly—or even color after they've had a baby. These changes are mainly due to hormone fluctuations, but may take some getting used to.

If Your Hair Is Thin or Limp

Don't pull your hair directly back into a tight ponytail. This severe-looking style will accentuate any thinning on the front of your hairline. It can also create breakage at the scalp and underneath the ponytail band, which won't help matters any. If you want to put your hair back—always a convenient option when you're short on time for showering and styling—try a loose ponytail or bun with soft pieces pulled out at the front. Use a volumizing shampoo to give your hair as much fullness as you can. Blowing your hair dry, especially upside down, is a good way to blast volume into it as it dries.

If Your Hair Is Coarse, Frizzy, or Dry

Switch to a moisturizing shampoo, and be sure to condition your hair frequently. Consider using a deep-conditioning rinse or mask once a week. Frizziness is caused by parched hair sucking the humidity out of the air. It can help to use a product that helps seal in your hair's natural moisture and keep out humidity. Try a leave-in frizz treatment when your hair is damp from the shower, and then finish up with a smoothing serum when it's dry. Don't pile on too many products, though—that'll just leave your hair looking weighed down. Dry, frizzy hair is made worse by heat, so don't overuse the hair dryer, or the straightening or curling iron.

Am I Balding?

Sometime around the third or fourth month postpartum, some women notice that their hair—which may have become quite thick and full during pregnancy—starts to fall out at a faster-than-normal rate. The natural shift in hormones that happens around this time triggers the hair to go from a growth phase, which it's in all during pregnancy, to a shedding phase. A normal, nonpregnant, nonpostpartum woman loses about 100 hairs a day, but a postpartum woman might lose three or four times that much. You might notice it everywhere—on your clothes, in your hairbrush, clogging up the shower drain. You may even notice some thinning near your temples and the front of your hairline. Don't worry—most of the time this hair loss is completely normal and will let up before you find yourself shopping for hairpieces.

Make an appointment to get a haircut sometime around the third or fourth month postpartum. You might be starting to feel frumpy if you haven't had your hair done since before the baby was born, and the haircut will be a nice pick-me-up. Plus, you can discuss any changes to your hair's texture or volume with your stylist, and she can recommend cuts and styles that will work best with your new hair and new lifestyle.

The Six-week Checkup

UNLESS YOU'VE HAD A home birth or birth-center birth, once you go home from the hospital you won't see your doctor or midwife again for six weeks. The six-week checkup is an opportunity for your care provider to monitor how you're healing from birth and to make sure you're adjusting well emotionally and physically to your new role as a mother. It's also a chance for you to ask your care provider questions about anything that might concern you, from bleeding, to sex, to diet and exercise, to breastfeeding.

What to Expect

At your visit, your care provider will check your weight and blood pressure. She'll check your abdomen to make sure there's no tenderness or unusual masses or lumps. She'll also examine your breasts and inspect your perineum to see that any tears, stitches, or abrasions are healing properly.

Your doctor or midwife may also do an internal exam to feel your uterus and ovaries and inspect your vaginal muscle tone, checking for pelvic floor damage or prolapse. Some care providers perform rectal exams as part of the six-week checkup, too.

Discussing Your Physical Recovery

If you have concerns over how quickly you're recovering, tell your care provider. By the six-week checkup, you should be feeling pretty good. Lingering soreness, extreme fatigue, or bleeding that hasn't stopped, or has stopped and started up again, should all be discussed. Also, be sure to tell her if you're having any trouble with nursing or if you've experienced any nipple infections, persistent painful nursing, clogged ducts, or other breast issues. She may be able to help you troubleshoot your nursing habits and see if positioning, pressure from your bra or clothing, or some other issue is causing problems.

Essential

You may need a Pap smear as part of your regular well-woman care during this visit, or to follow up on an abnormal result you had during pregnancy. Abnormal Pap smears are fairly common during pregnancy, and often the postpartum follow-up test will be normal. You may want to wait until three months postpartum to have your Pap done. Results will be more accurate, and you will likely be more ready for the speculum!

At this point your doctor or midwife will probably give you the go-ahead to start a fitness program. If you have any specific questions about diet, weight loss, or exercise, ask them during your visit.

Discussing Emotional Issues

If you're feeling sadness, anxiety, or another emotion that worries you, discuss it with your doctor or midwife. Some weepiness may be normal, but if you're experiencing something more serious, your care provider will want to know about it and may be able to help you. See Chapter 15 for more information about treating postpartum depression and other mood disorders.

Sex, Breastfeeding, and Birth Control

Your doctor or midwife will probably give you clearance to start having sex again at this point if everything's healing normally. Even if you aren't having a period yet, you may still be fertile during this time, so you should be thinking about birth control. Depending on your personal and religious beliefs, you may want to space your children closely, or rely on breastfeeding or other natural methods for child spacing. Or you may not be sure if you want more children, want to have kids a few years apart, or know for certain your family is complete. You should know about the options available to you so that, no matter what your family preferences and needs are, you'll feel prepared to resume your sex life.

If you're breastfeeding, your chances of conceiving again are already going to be reduced for a while. If your baby is exclusively nursing, nurses at least every four hours, doesn't rely on a pacifier for much of his sucking needs, and your period hasn't come back, your chances of getting pregnant in the first six months postpartum are around 2 percent; in other words, this lactational amenorrhea method (LAM) is more effective than many other methods of birth control. That's because the hormones released during frequent, exclusive nursing can keep you from ovulating and returning to fertility.

 Fact

It's important to keep nursing at night if you're relying on LAM as birth control. The hormones that cause fertility are most abundant at night, so you'll need to keep creating the fertility-suppressing hormones released during breastfeeding at night as well.

After your baby is six months old, your chances of getting pregnant go back up, even if you haven't had a period yet and are still nursing a lot. You won't always be warned by a period before you start ovulating, so don't rely on your first period as a sign that your fertility has returned. If you won't be breastfeeding, you'll need to think about contraception before the first time you have sex postpartum.

Mothers who aren't nursing at all can be fertile during even the earliest postpartum weeks and have even been known to be pregnant already by the six-week postpartum checkup! If you're bottle feeding or supplementing breastfeeding with formula, or if your nursing baby sleeps long stretches at night, frequently sucks a pacifier, is older than six months, eats solid foods, or regularly goes longer than four hours between feedings, the LAM method may be ineffective or less effective for you, and you should use another form of contraceptive if you want to prevent pregnancy.

Barrier Methods

Barrier methods of contraception literally block sperm from entering your cervix and causing pregnancy. Barrier methods can be a good choice while breastfeeding because they won't interfere with milk supply.

Male Condoms

Latex condoms are easy to find, relatively inexpensive, and protect against both pregnancy and sexually transmitted infections (STIs), which is important if you or your partner are not monogamous or have recently been with other partners. When they are used correctly every time, about three percent of women using them will become pregnant in a year. When your vaginal tissues are still tender, you may find that certain types of condoms—like the ribbed variety—create too much friction and are uncomfortable. You'll want to be sure to use plenty of water-based lubricant if you are experiencing uncomfortable dryness or friction with condoms. Some women are sensitive to latex or the spermicides used on some condoms, which can lead to itching, burning, and redness. If you or your partner is allergic or sensitive to latex, you can try a condom made of polyurethane.

Female Condoms

The female condom, also called the vaginal contraceptive pouch, is a relatively new option. It's a sheath inserted into the woman, lining the entire vagina with polyurethane, and held in place by soft, flexible rings at either end. The female condom is about 95 percent effective, meaning that when used correctly, about five women out of 100 will become pregnant in a year. Since it covers not only the entire inside of the vagina but also the vaginal opening, it can also protect against STIs. You can use an oil-based lubricant with the female condom, since it won't affect the polyurethane, but you shouldn't use female and male condoms together. The friction can cause the male condom to come off, or the female condom to slip to the side or tear. Female condoms are more expensive than male condoms and may be more difficult to find. Inserting and using the female condom may take some practice, and you might find that the ring that fits close to your cervix causes some irritation.

 Alert

Never use an oil- or petroleum-based lubricant, like a massage oil, Vaseline, or hand lotion, with a latex condom, since any oils can break down the latex in the condom. On the other hand, polyurethane condoms can be used with oil-based lubricants.

Diaphragm

The diaphragm is a small rubber or silicone device shaped like a dome, filled with spermicidal jelly or cream, and then inserted into the vagina, blocking the cervix, before sex. The spermicide is used to kill any sperm that may work their way in around the rim. Though certain cervical infections such as gonorrhea, chlamydia, or HPV are less likely to be transmitted if you're using a diaphragm, this method isn't considered effective protection against STIs.

Sometimes, you can get a diaphragm at your six-week postpartum visit, but you may have to wait longer if your vaginal muscle tone isn't strong enough yet to ensure a good fit. By three months postpartum, most women have sufficient vaginal muscle tone to use a diaphragm. In the meantime, you can use another form of birth control if you want to resume sex, or you can rely on lactational amenorrhea if you meet the guidelines given previously.

If you're ready to be fitted for a diaphragm, your care provider will perform a pelvic exam to estimate your size, then try several sizes of fitting rings until she finds the one that's the right size for your body. Your care provider can also show you how to use the diaphragm. Since they're available by prescription only, she can either give you one in her office or write you a prescription to pick one up at a pharmacy.

 Question

How effective is a diaphragm at preventing pregnancy?
When it's used correctly, the diaphragm is about 94 percent effective. Using the diaphragm without spermicide reduces its effectiveness. If you're not comfortable with a 6 percent failure rate, you may use the diaphragm in conjunction with another method, like condoms.

You'll need to buy spermicide that's meant to be used with the diaphragm, but you can find this over the counter, usually near the condoms, in most drugstores. If you or your partner is sensitive to spermicides, the diaphragm isn't a great method for you, since using it without spermicide makes it much less effective.

If you opt to use a diaphragm, you can put it in up to six hours before having sex, and you must leave it in at least six hours after having sex so that the spermicide can kill all the sperm. It can be tricky the first few times you put it in, but most women get the hang of it quickly. The diaphragm may not be for you if you're uncomfortable feeling inside your own body, since you'll need to be able to make sure it's inserted deeply into your vagina and covering your cervix.

After a few tries you will become familiar with the way your cervix feels, and it will become easier to tell when the diaphragm is positioned correctly.

 Alert

Even if you've used a diaphragm in the past, it's imperative that you get refitted after giving birth. Pregnancy and birth can change the size and shape of your cervix, even if you had a c-section.

If your diaphragm is made of latex rubber, make sure not to use an oil-based lubricant with it like petroleum jelly, baby oil, or mineral oil, since it can weaken the rubber. Water-based lubricants, like KY jelly or mist, are fine. If your diaphragm is made of silicone, you can use any kind of lubricant. You can leave the diaphragm in up to twenty-four hours at a time, but it's better to remove it six to eight hours after having sex. If you leave it in longer, you may risk developing toxic shock syndrome, a rare but very serious illness. You'll also need to regularly check your diaphragm for signs of wear and tear, clean it carefully after each use, and store it away from heat, moisture, and light to make sure the rubber doesn't break down. If you lose or gain a significant amount of weight, have an abortion or miscarriage, or undergo pelvic surgery, you'll have to be refitted for a new diaphragm.

Cervical Cap

In some ways, a cervical cap is very similar to a diaphragm: it works as a barrier method, blocking sperm from reaching your cervix. Your care provider will fit you for it at or after your six-week checkup, then show you how to insert it and care for it. You'll use the cervical cap with spermicidal jelly or cream made specially for use with a cervical cap.

A cervical cap can be inserted up to twenty-four hours before intercourse, allowing for a fair amount of spontaneity. You'll need to leave the cap in place for at least eight hours after sex, but you can leave it in much longer than the diaphragm (up to forty-eight hours). You won't be able to use a cervical cap during your period or if you have a yeast or other vaginal infection. Like with the diaphragm, oil-based lubricants or medications like yeast infection cream can damage the latex. If you're allergic to latex or spermicides, a cervical cap isn't a good option for you.

 Fact

> While the cervical cap's effectiveness is sometimes rated as highly as that of the diaphragm, being a mom appears to make the cap less effective. Since your cervix may have changed shape after giving birth, the cap may not be able to effectively block the opening.

The cervical cap can get more easily knocked out of place during sex than a diaphragm. And, like the diaphragm, the cervical cap can cause vaginal irritation and increases the risk of urinary tract infection and pelvic infections, including toxic shock syndrome. If you have a cervical cap, you'll need to be refitted every time you have another baby, or if you miscarry or have an abortion.

Spermicides

As the name suggests, spermicides are chemicals that kill sperm. They're available over the counter and come in several forms—cream, jelly, foam, and dissolvable film, with a variety of application methods. They can be used alone or with diaphragms or condoms, which will make them more effective. Spermicides can be messy and may cause irritation.

Used alone, spermicides aren't considered very reliable forms of birth control, but they can greatly increase the effectiveness of other methods, like the male or female condom. Many women and men find that they're sensitive or allergic to spermicides. You may also find that you have a reaction to certain spermicidal products but not to others.

 Alert

Spermicides containing nonoxynol-9 can change the pH balance in your vagina and lead to urinary tract infections, so you may want to seek out a spermicide that contains octoxynol-9 instead.

IUD

The intrauterine device, or IUD, is a T-shaped piece of plastic or copper placed inside your uterus by your doctor or midwife. Some IUDs also release the hormone progestin, which makes it more effective at preventing pregnancy. Since the IUD releases the hormone directly into the uterine lining, not much of it gets into your bloodstream, so the IUD may be a good choice for you even if you've disliked the side effects of hormonal contraceptives in the past. You'll want to wait at least six weeks after having a baby before having an IUD placed, since the uterine cramping that happens after giving birth can cause your body to expel the device if it's inserted too early. Also, inserting the hormonal IUD before your milk supply is well established could cause your production to be diminished.

Hormonal Contraceptives

Hormonal contraceptives include the Pill, the mini-pill, the patch, the ring, implants, and injections. Some hormonal contraceptives include estrogen, some contain a combination of estrogen and progesterone (progestin), and others, like the mini-pill, contain progestin only. If you're not breastfeeding, you'll need to start a hormonal method quickly: Non-nursing mothers can start ovulating again as soon as forty-five days after the birth of their baby, and hormonal forms of contraception can take a few weeks to start working. Talk to your care provider about the contraception that will fit your lifestyle best, and what kind of reliable backup method you can use until the hormones begin protecting you from pregnancy.

When it comes to hormone-based contraceptives, nursing mothers will want to follow a few rules. First, avoid estrogen, which has been shown to decrease the quality and quantity of breastmilk, for the first six months of nursing. Second, wait until at least six weeks, when your milk supply is well established, to start taking hormonal contraceptives. And third, start with the lowest effective dose available. There are several progestin-only forms of birth control you may want to try.

Progestin-only Pill

Also called the mini-pill, the progestin-only is considered safe for your baby and is reported not to affect milk supply. It's important to note that even though experts say that the progestin won't reduce the amount of milk you produce, anecdotally, a small number of women say that they feel progestin does affect their milk supply. There are also other side effects that are associated with any kind of hormonal contraceptive, including nausea, headaches, weight gain, and a decreased sex drive. Like the combination or estrogen-only pill, you shouldn't take the mini-pill if you're a smoker over the age of thirty-five, and there are certain health conditions that can make taking any hormonal contraceptive dangerous. Be sure to discuss your health history thoroughly with your care provider before starting on any kind of hormonal contraceptive.

When you take the mini-pill, you'll want to remember a few key things: first, timing is much more important than it is with the combination pill. You'll need to be sure to take your pill at about the same time every day, which isn't always easy when you've got a new baby to care for. Also, there are no sugar pills, also known as placebos, in a pack of progestin-only pills (POPs)—every pill contains the same amount of medication, so you'll need to take a pill every day until the pack is finished, then start a new pack right away. Also, if you have enjoyed the way a combination pill evens out your menstrual cycles in the past, be aware that the mini-pill won't do that—if you're naturally inclined to have irregular or heavy periods, they will stay irregular and heavy while on the mini-pill. You also won't be able to plan or predict when your period is going to be—it could come at any point in the pack, unlike with the combination pill.

 Fact

> While the progestin-only pill (mini-pill) is slightly less effective than combination pills, the added protection breastfeeding provides generally makes the mini-pill very successful at preventing pregnancy in a frequently breastfeeding mother. Once your baby is eating a lot of solids and nursing less, you may want to switch to the combination pill.

The Shot

Another form of progestin-only hormonal contraception is the Depo-Provera shot. There are several benefits to the shot: You won't have to remember to take a pill every day, and it lasts twelve weeks. The downside is that if you change your mind, don't like the way the hormones make you feel, or find that the progestin does in fact affect your milk supply, you're stuck with it for three months until the shot wears off.

Implants

The contraceptive implant, known as Norplant, is another progestin-only option. Norplant consists of six matchstick-sized rubber implants, which are placed under the skin of your upper arm (your care provider will numb your arm first). The risks of becoming pregnant while on Norplant are very low, and it's effective for up to five years. But as with any hormonal birth control, you may not like the way you feel when on Norplant, and you'll have to make another trip to your doctor's office if you want to have it removed.

Other Hormonal Methods

Lunelle, the monthly birth-control shot; Ortho Evra, the birth-control patch; and NuvaRing, the birth-control ring, all contain estrogen and may cause a drop in milk supply. If you're nursing, it's best to wait until your baby is at least six months old and eating solid foods before beginning to use one of these forms of birth control. If you have experienced problems with your milk supply in the past, you may be susceptible to lowered milk production even after six months.

Emergency Contraception

The FDA recently approved the over-the-counter sale of Plan B, an emergency contraception that contains only progestin. Contrary to some misconceptions, the morning-after pill is not the same as the early-abortion pill RU-486. Plan B works by delivering a higher dosage of the same hormones present in birth-control pills, preventing your body from releasing an egg, or if your egg has already been released, preventing it from becoming fertilized or attaching to the uterine wall, the same way a regular birth-control pill functions. If you are already pregnant, the morning-after pill will not affect your pregnancy or cause you to miscarry.

Essential

If you experience decreased milk supply after taking progestin pills, you may experience a supply problem after taking Plan B. Get plenty of rest, drink lots of fluids, and nurse more often.

Keep in mind that emergency contraception is meant to be just that—used in an emergency, in case you forget your regular birth control, or another form of birth control fails. While Plan B is considered safe for nursing mothers, it can cause headaches, nausea, and abdominal pain, and you should take it very soon after having unprotected sex—within seventy-two hours, but the earlier the better—for it to be effective.

Natural Family Planning

If you don't want to use barrier or hormonal contraception for personal, medical, or religious reasons, but do not want to start having more children right away, natural family planning (NFP) may be a good option for you. NFP requires dedication and consistency, since the method requires being very in tune with one's ovulation symptoms, keeping detailed charts, and refraining from sexual intercourse for nearly two weeks out of the month. It can be tricky to become accustomed to the method, but once you have it down, NFP shouldn't take more than a minute or two out of each day. Many women enjoy being more in tune with their body's fertility signals, and men can take an active role in this form of birth control by helping the woman chart her cycles.

Choosing a Method

There are two methods of natural family planning (NFP), also called the fertility awareness method (FAM): the ovulation method and the symptothermal method. With the ovulation method, also called the mucus-only method, a woman checks her cervical mucus daily to assess where she is in her menstrual cycle. Using the symptothermal method, the woman charts both her mucus and her daily temperature, which rises during ovulation.

With either method, the couple must refrain from having unprotected sex between the period a week before and three days after the woman ovulates. When used correctly, NFP's success rates are quite good—only a 3 percent failure rate for the mucus-only method, and a 2 percent failure rate for the symptothermal method.

L. Essential

If you decide to use natural family planning as a method of birth control, it's very important that you receive training from a qualified instructor or closely follow a manual that teaches you what signs to look for and how to chart them. The Couple to Couple League may be a good place to start; its Web site is ⌕*www.ccli.org.*

Rhythm Method

You may have heard of the calendar, or rhythm method, which is a less effective form of natural family planning where the woman evaluates her cycle over several months, then, on the assumption that ovulation occurs at the midpoint of the cycle, refrains from having sex in the week before and the three days after that date. But not everybody ovulates on exactly the same point of every cycle, so this method isn't nearly as exact as the symptothermal or even the mucus-only method. Still, with a failure rate of 9 percent, it may be a risk you're comfortable taking if you don't mind having closely spaced children and are willing to let nature have a large say in when you become pregnant again.

Breastfeeding and NFP

Be aware that your ovulation signs may not be predictable or apparent while you're nursing, and your periods may not become regular for some time while you're breastfeeding. If you're nursing, it's especially important that your instructor or book specifically addresses using NFP while breastfeeding.

Sterilization

In addition to the reversible methods of birth control listed above, undergoing surgery to become infertile is an option for either you or your partner. Different forms of sterilization follow.

Tubal Ligation

Tubal ligation, also known as getting your "tubes tied," is a procedure in which the surgeon creates a surgical incision below your navel and either ties off or cauterizes your fallopian tubes. This procedure can be done within a day or so after you give birth, before you leave the hospital—in fact, it can be easier for the surgeon to perform this procedure shortly after the birth of a baby because the position of your uterus makes it easier for the surgeon to reach your fallopian tubes. If you have a c-section birth, the tubal ligation can be done at the same time as the surgery before your doctor closes up your abdominal incision.

Tubal ligation is very effective and is one of the most popular forms of contraception in the United States. But there are health risks involved with any kind of surgery, and tubal ligation is considered a more invasive and risky surgery than male sterilization, or vasectomy. Also, it's very difficult to reverse the procedure once it's done, and is considered a permanent means of birth control. You'll need to very carefully consider whether you'll want to have more children before you plan a tubal ligation. If you've had a stressful pregnancy or had a difficult birth experience, you may think you won't ever want to have more children, but it's possible you may change your mind later. Unless you are absolutely sure that there are no circumstances under which you might want to get pregnant again, you may want to wait until your life has settled down a little bit before deciding to have a tubal ligation. Your care provider can help you decide on a method of contraception to use in the meanwhile.

Vasectomy

Vasectomy isn't for everyone, but it is a very safe and effective option for many. It is far less invasive and risky than female sterilization, not to mention less expensive. During a vasectomy, a doctor will make a small incision on each side of the scrotum, snip the vas deferens tubes, then tie them off or cauterize them. The procedure should take less than an hour and only requires a local anesthetic and no hospitalization. It can take a while for the man's semen to become free of sperm, so his doctor will probably ask him to provide some sperm-free semen samples before he's given the all-clear to have unprotected sex, which can take up to three months. In the meanwhile, you'll have to abstain from sex or use another form of birth control. If you're absolutely sure neither of you want to have more children, you can arrange for your husband to have the procedure early in the postpartum period or while you're pregnant, though some doctors will refuse to perform the procedure on a man whose wife is pregnant.

L. Essential

Though the vasectomy procedure is safe and simple, many men are a little queasy at the thought of any cutting in "that area." Though some women are able to use the "Hey, I gave birth, now it's your turn" line of reasoning to convince their men to go under the knife, it doesn't always work. Some men, however, are relieved by being able to exert such control over their own fertility and will gladly—or at least resolutely—volunteer for the procedure.

If you and your husband both know you're done having children and you really want him to consider vasectomy, but he gives a knee-jerk veto, try playing up the benefits. The two of you will be able to enjoy much more freedom and spontaneity in your sex life; you won't have to worry about hormones that may give you mood swings, or barrier methods that can reduce both your enjoyment; and most of all, eliminating the fear of getting pregnant again may make you both feel a little sexier. He may just see things your way.

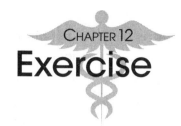

CHAPTER 12

Exercise

DON'T WORRY THAT YOU have to train for a triathalon with your baby strapped to your back to reap the rewards of exercise. Whether you're walking, dancing, or taking a yoga class for new moms, any movement will tone your muscles, burn calories, and build endurance. Research suggests that new mothers who exercise are often happier and better adjusted to parenthood. And exercise will help increase your energy levels, can help make your sleep patterns more regular, and in general can help you be happier and healthier.

Are You Ready?

Experts differ on when it's okay to start a postpartum exercise routine. Many suggest waiting until six weeks postpartum, but research also shows that starting certain exercises much earlier than that can be both safe and beneficial.

Before you start doing any abdominal exercises, you'll need to make sure you don't have a diastasis, or separation of your abdominal muscles. These are common and will usually heal spontaneously, but if you begin exercising your abdominal muscles too hard before a separation heals, you may risk injuring the muscles.

To see if you have a separation, lie flat on your back with your knees bent, and place your left hand just above your bellybutton. Take a breath, and as you exhale, lift your head and shoulders off the floor and begin to pick your right hand up off the floor, too. You will feel your abdominal muscles tighten and will probably notice a gap between the muscles. If the gap is more than three fingers wide, hold off on doing crunches or sit-ups or other strenuous abdominal exercise until the gap shrinks to smaller than a finger's width.

 Question

I delivered my baby via cesarean section. When can I start exercising?
Generally, mothers who've had c-sections are advised to wait six to eight weeks before starting an exercise program. Talk to your doctor or midwife at your six-week checkup and get clearance before you start exercising.

Finding Time

In addition to physical constraints, one of the biggest obstacles to starting a postpartum exercise routine is finding the time for one. If you've gotten the idea that an exercise routine has to include hours of working out and you can't ever skip a day, you'll probably be even more intimidated. Don't worry—you don't have to be an Olympian to get back in shape. In fact, it's better to take it slow so your new body can adjust to the increased activity.

Any amount of exercise is better than no exercise at all. If all you can manage right now is getting out for a walk every other day, embrace it. If you go out for a jog with your baby and find that you have to stop every ten minutes to feed or comfort him, that's OK—exercise doesn't have to be continuous to count. Try not to judge your efforts or get frustrated if you don't feel like you're doing "enough." As your baby gets older, it will become easier to squeeze in longer workouts.

If You're Breastfeeding

Contrary to what you may have heard, nursing moms can exercise safely. It's true that lactic acid, which is released by your muscles while exercising, can get into your breastmilk, but the lactic acid is safe for your baby. If you nurse your baby immediately after exercising, it may slightly change the taste of your milk, and some babies may reject the saltier flavor. You can avoid this problem by nursing your baby right before you exercise; by the time you feed him again, the lactic acid will most likely be gone from your milk. This will also help keep you more comfortable, since your breasts will be lighter while you're exercising.

Exercises for the Early Weeks

While you probably won't want to start running miles a day before your body has had a chance to heal completely, most moms can start doing some gentle stretching and toning exercises from the second week on. There are even exercises you can do in bed or on the sofa.

Kegel, Kegel, Kegel

The most important exercise you can do in the early postpartum weeks are Kegels. To help your pelvic floor heal, you need to get the blood flowing to this area and tone up the muscles. (See Chapter 3 for instructions on how to do Kegel exercises.) Do Kegels several times a day for best results. At first, it may help to lie on your back and apply pressure to your perineum to help you "find" the muscles, but eventually you should be able to perform Kegels whenever you have a spare moment, whether you're on a long car ride or in line at the bank.

Back, Neck, and Shoulders

You may find that your back, neck, and shoulder muscles become sore from holding and looking down at your baby. If you have this problem, several times a day, stretch your arms above your head and sit up as straight as you can, and then lie on the floor with your arms above your head. From this position, pull your knees to your chest and rock back and forth, allowing the floor to give your spine a massage. Remember to pull your legs up one at a time to your chest. Lifting them together at the same time puts pressure on the diastasis.

Pelvic or Hip Tilts

Lying on your back with your knees bent and your feet flat on the floor, tilt your pelvis upward so that your tailbone moves toward your bellybutton. Your hips should remain on the floor—movement should be only in your pelvis. When you've tilted up a few inches, tighten your rear end, hold for a second, then release and repeat six to eight times. You can also squeeze your tummy muscles tight and release a few times for more toning while lying on your back, standing, or on your hands and knees. This will gently tone your abdominal muscles.

Head and Shoulder Raises

Continue to lie in the same position as you were for the pelvic tilts. Take a deep breath. As you exhale, tighten your tummy muscles, tilt your pelvis forward so that your back presses into the floor, and raise your head and shoulders a little (don't overdo it!). Lower to the floor gently and repeat six to eight times. Check for abdominal separation—if you can feel it, it's too much.

Gentle Aerobic Exercise

You can also start walking outside or on a treadmill, swimming, or doing low-impact aerobic exercise as soon as you feel up to it after giving birth, but take it easy in the first few weeks. It might not take a lot to tire you out.

On the other hand, many women get a psychological and physiological boost from exercise, and find that it increases energy levels and improves mood. Still other women physically need exercise, sometimes vigorous exercise, to maintain a sense of well-being. If you want to go back to a strenuous workout routine soon after giving birth, talk to your doctor or midwife about it. He or she may have no problem with the idea as long as you are healing well from birth.

No matter what kind of exercise you start doing, listen to your body. Stop if you feel exhausted, in pain, dizzy, or weak, or if your lochia returns or increases after slowing or stopping.

Alert

Remember relaxin, the hormone that made your joints and ligaments loose during pregnancy? You'll continue to produce it for a few months after giving birth, so be careful—it's easy to overstretch and hurt yourself during the postpartum period.

Taking It Up a Notch

Once you're feeling up to more energetic activity, you can participate in a number of other great forms of postpartum exercise. Some of these include brisk walking, swimming, biking, yoga, and Pilates. And if you have clearance from your care practitioner, you may even be able to resume your prepregnancy exercise routine.

Brisk Walking

Walking is a great exercise for postpartum moms. It's easy, it's low impact, it's adaptable to your energy and fitness level, it's free, and you can do it with your baby in a front- or backpack, sling, or stroller. Walking improves your circulation, can get a sluggish digestive system moving, and can be a wonderful way to relieve stress, get fresh air, clear your head, and improve your mood. Often, even the fussiest babies will calm down as soon as you step outside, so many new moms take to going for long walks just to keep the baby happy.

The trick to turning a gentle stroll into a workout is picking up the pace. When you first start walking, choose a pace that's brisk but doesn't tire you out right away. As you build up your endurance and pass the six-week postpartum point, though, cranking your speed up a few notches will burn more calories. Warm up first with five minutes or so of slow walking, marching in place, or lunges. Once you can walk for twenty minutes or longer without tiring out, you can increase your speed so that you're walking a mile in fifteen minutes.

Experts suggest exercising three to five times a week for thirty minutes or more, but any amount of exercise is better than no exercise; even a daily ten- or fifteen-minute walk will deliver health results and can improve your outlook. When it's raining or snowing outside, try the local mall or see if your community center has an indoor track.

Swimming

Swimming is another great low-impact exercise that burns calories, increases stamina, and gets the heart and lungs functioning more efficiently. Since you won't be able to use tampons during the postpartum period, you'll probably have to wait until your lochia has stopped before you can begin or resume swimming. Heading to the pool isn't quite as mom- and baby-friendly as walking—unless you have your own pool, you'll have to work around the schedule at your community pool, athletic club, or YMCA, and you'll probably have to wait until your partner is available to watch the baby or use some kind of child care. Many gyms and YMCAs offer child care, but most won't let you start using it until your baby is at least six weeks old.

Biking

Riding a bike is gentle on the knees and other joints, and if you have a bike trailer or baby seat, you can take your little one along. It may be awhile before your perineum is able to handle a bike seat, however—sitting on a bike could cause or exacerbate soreness and swelling if you don't wait until you're completely healed.

Yoga

Yoga is a gentle way to get your body moving again, relieve some of the stress of new motherhood, gain more energy, and regain strength and flexibility. You may also find that yoga provides a way to tap into the calmness that might be hiding beneath a surface of frazzled nerves and spit-up!

Yoga classes designed specifically for new mothers are becoming more and more popular. Most allow you to bring your baby with you and will incorporate him into the practice, allowing you to come and go as necessary to feed, change, or comfort him. Postpartum yoga classes usually focus on gently re-aligning the postpartum body, particularly by strengthening the abdominal and pelvic muscles after childbirth. A mom-baby yoga class can also provide you with a ready-made community of new mothers, and you won't have to worry about finding a babysitter.

L. Essential

Check your local community center, health club, or yoga studio to see if there's a postpartum yoga class available. If there isn't, you can try following a postpartum yoga program from a book or magazine, CD, or DVD.

Serious yoginis may be frustrated by the slower pace and beginning level of some postpartum yoga classes, as well as the fact that mom-and-baby classes are full of interruptions! If you have been practicing yoga for some time, you may be more satisfied in a more advanced class. Still, even if the postpartum class is a little less challenging than you'd like, you may find that you enjoy the opportunity to chat with other moms. If you decide to take a regular class that's not specifically for postpartum women, be sure you let the instructor know that you've recently had a baby—she may suggest that you skip or modify certain poses.

Pilates

Pilates focuses on strengthening your abdominal and back muscles, what's known as your "core." This makes it particularly well suited to rebuilding abdominal, back, and pelvic-floor muscles that have been left saggy or strained from pregnancy. Pilates instructors emphasize good posture and give extremely detailed instructions, helping you fine-tune your form throughout the process.

Since Pilates exercises are so specific, taking a class through your local health club or YMCA may be the best option. There are also books and DVDs that lay out postpartum Pilates programs you can do at home. If you take a class that's not specifically geared toward postpartum women, be sure to let the instructor know you've had a baby so she can show you how to do the exercises without injuring your abdominal muscles.

Your Usual Routine

If your prebaby workout routine included off-road biking, dancing, kickboxing, running, martial arts, horseback riding, or other vigorous exercise, your doctor or midwife will probably give you the go-ahead to start up again by your sixth week postpartum (maybe a little longer if you had a c-section). Sometimes athletes have a hard time adjusting to their recovering body's limitations, and you may feel frustrated that you can't do as much as you were able to before. Try to remember that it will take a little while for your body to return to the condition it was in before, but as you get stronger and your baby gets older, you'll gradually be able to incorporate your sport back into your life more and more.

Working Out with Baby In-arms

Walking and jogging can be done easily enough with baby in a stroller, but bad weather and older kids at home can make it difficult to get out for a walk or run. Many new moms are stumped when it comes to how to exercise at home with a baby. Not all infants are content to lie next to you or lounge in a bouncy seat while you're exercising, and baby's naptime should be your resting time, too.

Exercising with your baby in a sling or front-pack carrier can be a lifesaver for moms of babies who are happiest when snuggled close. You can exercise with your baby in-arms as long as you follow these safety guidelines:

- Any fluid, nonjouncing exercise that you can do with a baby on your chest can be safe as long as you make sure to support your baby's head and neck and stay upright.
- You shouldn't do any kind of jiggling or bouncing motion, like running, with your baby in a sling or front-pack carrier. Carriers and slings don't provide the support and shock absorption that a jogging stroller would, and it's easy to injure a baby's spinal cord from too much jouncing.
- Choose slow, steady movements like plies and lunges when you have your baby in-arms. To do these safely, you should make sure your back stays straight (don't bend forward with your baby in a sling or carrier). Keep one hand on your baby, and use the wall or the back of a chair or sofa for support.
- For arm and ab exercises, you can actually use your baby for resistance—if he or she is willing and not too heavy. You can do bicep curls with your baby being the "dumbbell," or do crunches with your baby reclining against your lap at a 45-degree angle.

If you're unsure how a particular exercise will affect your baby, always ask your care practitioner for guidance before giving it a try. You'll get more out of your workout if you go into it with all the information you need.

Getting the Right Stuff

Depending on what kind of exercise you want to do, you might need a piece or two of specialized equipment. You may already have the basics, such as sneakers and workout clothing, but it's probably a good idea to invest in some new gear to help you feel more comfortable during those first weeks. The following sections cover a few items you may need and offer suggestions for where to find them.

Good Shoes

This is a must-have if you'll be jogging or performing another higher-impact activity because you can injure yourself wearing ill-fitting shoes that don't offer adequate support. You may also find that you need more supportive shoes than you did prepregnancy, or that the style of shoes you used to wear no longer work as well. During pregnancy, your feet may have gone through a variety of changes—they might be longer, wider, or flatter now. Your gait may even have changed. Shop around at discount shoe warehouses—often they offer last year's favorites at bargain-basement prices

Jogging Strollers, Bike Trailers, or Bike Seats

These items can make your life much easier. Bike trailers and jogging strollers provide the baby with support and shock absorption, and jogging strollers are generally easier to push on all kinds of terrain than regular strollers. These items can be expensive, but check with your church or parenting community before plunking down big bucks for a new model. Often, people give these items away, or sell them for a song and a dance. Also check your local Freecycle listings (*www.freecycle.com*) or Craigslist (*www.craigslist.org*), your community and daily newspaper want ads, your grocery store bulletin boards, and consignment and thrift stores for gently used bargains. If you like to bike and run or walk, look for a bike trailer that doubles as a jogging stroller, which can save closet space and money.

Apparel

Don't underestimate the importance of a good, supportive running bra. Your breasts may be denser and heavier than they were prepregnancy, even if they aren't a lot larger. A bra that keeps your breasts in place without squeezing or compressing milk ducts is essential to your comfort (and to keep your breast tissue from breaking down and causing more sagging).

Home-exercise Equipment

A piece of home-exercise equipment you'll actually use can be a money saver, but the key words here are "you'll actually use." Before you invest the big bucks in a system that can tone your butt, thighs, and belly in eight easy moves, spend a few dollars on a set of 5-pound dumbbells, and a book or DVD that walks you through simple weight-training workouts. If you don't ever use the dumbbells, you probably won't be inclined to use the all-in-one system, either.

One exception to that may be a treadmill or exercise bike. If you love to walk, run, or bike, but the weather makes it difficult some or all of the time, these items can be a nice compromise. You can jump on the treadmill when your baby's napping or put him in front of you in a bouncy seat and sing or talk to him as you run.

Getting Support

It's not always easy to convince your partner to help you when it comes to establishing an exercise program. Even though men want their wives to be happy and healthy and are often eager for her to return to her prebaby shape and energy—not to mention sex drive—men don't always see the link between those things and exercise. Talk to your partner about your needs, and ask him to help make it possible for you to get the exercise that will make both your lives better.

How Your Partner Can Help

Your partner may want to help but may be unsure of how to do it, so give him ideas. Figure out specific ways he can help you make exercise a part of your life. This could include him getting up a little earlier in the morning, taking over for you so that you can squeeze in a workout before he goes to work, making sure not to schedule any activities during your evening workout time, or even brainstorming ways to soothe a high-needs baby so that you feel comfortable stealing away for a workout.

If You Don't Have Support

Single mothers or those with partners who work long hours, who travel, or who are otherwise not available may have a harder time getting the exercise they want or need. For some moms, the answer may be as simple as accepting that, right now, caring for your baby trumps an organized exercise program. Those moms could try working in as much physical activity as possible: walking to the store instead of driving may not look like a workout, but it's still calorie-burning, body-strengthening exercise. Don't compare yourself to other moms and what they may seem to be accomplishing—their situation may be very different from yours. Try reaching out to other moms in the same boat; you can help one another and feel better about not having a partner's support. You might even be able to trade child care for each other's workout time.

Some moms who don't have a partner's support in exercise endeavors may feel a greater need for exercise, not just as an extra but as a necessary part of their everyday wellness. If you're one of these moms, you will probably have to work a little harder to incorporate exercise into your everyday life, but you'll be more motivated to do so, too.

Using Child Care

If your local health club or YMCA offers babysitting services, this can be a convenient way to get in a workout without worrying about having child care lined up. But the quality of these centers varies widely. Make sure yours is staffed by experienced child-care providers, has a low child-care provider ratio, and doesn't accept sick children. Also, you may feel more comfortable if your gym has some kind of notification system so that they can call you if your baby is hungry or inconsolable.

Getting Back to Your Normal Shape

How quickly will your belly look "normal" again? This depends on how much you gained during pregnancy, how many children you have, how much you exercise, and that one factor you have no control over—your genes. Even with regular exercise and a great diet, your postpartum "pooch" may never disappear completely. You may need to become accustomed to a new definition of "normal."

Remember, you can't spot tone. If you only do abdominal exercises but don't do any aerobic exercise, you'll just strengthen the muscles below the layer of fat on your belly. You may feel better, but you probably won't look much different. Combining strength training and toning exercises with aerobic activity like walking, running, biking, or swimming will give you more noticeable results.

CHAPTER 13

Weight Loss and Nutrition

NOW THAT YOUR BABY is born, you may expect all the extra weight you put on during pregnancy to disappear. But it takes nine months to put on your pregnancy weight, and you should give yourself at least that long to take it off. Instead of focusing on how much weight you can lose, it's much more important to make sure you're eating a healthy, well-balanced diet and getting plenty of the nutrients you need during the postpartum months.

Getting the Nutrition You Need

It's difficult and impractical to count every calorie and tally up the vitamins and minerals you're taking in all day—and besides that, it's unnecessary. Getting enough of the nutrients you'll need to keep healthy, whether you're nursing or not, is straightforward if you eat when you're hungry, and consume a healthy, balanced diet containing a variety of fruits and vegetables, whole grains, lean meats or another protein source, dairy products or another calcium source, and a small amount of healthy fat like the kind found in olive oil or fish.

Saturated fats, like those found in fat from animal sources and a few plant sources, can raise "bad" blood cholesterol and are linked to heart disease. Trans fats, which are found in many processed foods and oil described as "hydrogenated" or "partially hydrogenated," can be even less healthy. Many food manufacturers and even some fast-food restaurants are now eliminating trans fats from some of their products. Opt for trans-fat–free processed and prepared foods when you can get them, and when you're cooking, use healthier oils like olive or canola.

As with any other time, the best way to healthfully lose weight now is to think not in terms of dieting, but in terms of changing the way you eat. Chances are good there are some things you can improve about your diet without actually eating less.

L. Essential

You can cut back on your fat consumption if you normally eat a lot of it, but make sure you're still getting some healthy fats, like olive oil, avocado, fish, or canola oil, and enough protein—lean meats, low-fat dairy products, soy, lentils, and beans are good sources of protein.

Do you put butter on everything? Maybe you could trade that big dollop of butter on your bread for a little drizzle of flavored olive oil instead. Do you drink soda or sweetened tea or coffee drinks? You might be amazed at how many empty (non-nutritive) calories are in your habitual comfort beverage—a popular chocolate coffee drink at a nationwide chain java joint packs almost 300 calories, and that's when it's made with skim milk. Do you drink a glass of wine or beer with dinner several times a week? Not only are alcoholic drinks full of calories, but also they can decrease your body's ability to recognize signs of fullness, meaning you're more likely to overindulge.

Breastfeeding and Calorie Needs

Breastfeeding mothers need at least 1,500 to 1,800 calories just to function, with 1,500 being the absolute minimum amount you must take in. Research has shown that mothers who eat fewer than 1,500 calories a day experience a drop in milk supply. Many women will find that 1,500 calories aren't nearly enough to keep them feeling satisfied through a busy day of caring for an infant.

Fact

The resting metabolic rate for an average thirty-year-old woman who is 5 feet, 5 inches tall and weighs 135 pounds is 1,400 calories. That means that a woman of that age, height, and weight needs to consume 1,400 calories per day just to support her body's vital functions—nothing else.

You'll need 200 to 500 calories or more for breastfeeding. Add in the number of calories you'll burn just existing, and then consider that, as the mother of a small baby, you'll be doing a lot more than just existing, and you'll see that the "necessary" 1,500 calories is very much on the low end for most women.

Nutrition for Nursing Moms

If you already had a great diet before, you'll need to add one serving each of dairy, whole grains, fruit, and green vegetables now that you're breastfeeding. Nursing moms should eat at least seven servings of protein-rich foods per day, with at least one of these coming from a vegetable. Great sources of protein include lean meats and fish, milk and yogurt, nuts, beans, and legumes.

You'll need at least three servings of calcium-rich foods per day. The easiest way to get add calcium in your diet is probably by drinking milk, but you can also get calcium from sources like leafy green vegetables; yogurt and cheese; almonds; blackstrap molasses; shellfish; and calcium-enriched bread, orange juice, or cereal.

Reach for seven servings of grains per day. Look for labels that say "whole grain" or "whole wheat"; these tend to be far less processed and will deliver more fiber.

Veggies and fruits should be high on your list. You'll need a total of five or six per day. At least one should be rich in vitamin C, like citrus fruits, and another should be high in vitamin A, like carrots or sweet potatoes.

L. Essential

If you aren't absolutely sure you're diet is giving you the nutrients you need, continue taking your prenatal vitamin or start taking a multivitamin every day. You may also want to add an essential fatty acid, like fish-oil capsules or DHA supplements.

You should also consume some unsaturated fats, like the kind found in fish or fish oil supplements; nuts; seeds; avocados; and olive, canola, or soybean oil, each day. Remember, your body needs some fat to be healthy—just make sure you're getting mostly the good kind. Most of us already get enough omega-6 fatty acids, found in corn and safflower oil, for example, through the standard American diet, and too many omega-6 fatty acids can interfere with the balance between omega-3 and omega-6 acids that our bodies need to be healthy.

Special Diets and Breastfeeding

If you are a vegetarian or vegan for health or ethical reasons, you may wonder if you need to give up your diet in order to make healthy milk. But vegetarian and vegan diets can be healthy for both you and your baby as long as you take care to consume enough essential nutrients.

Vegetarians

Most experts agree that a vegetarian diet can be healthy for breastfeeding moms. If you eat animal protein like eggs, milk, cheese, or other dairy products, you're probably already getting enough calcium, zinc, and vitamin B-12.

Vegans

If you don't eat any animal products at all, you may need to be more vigilant about making sure you get enough calcium, zinc, B-12, and healthy fats, either by eating a diet naturally high in these nutrients, consuming fortified foods, or taking supplements. Most likely you were already careful to get all the nutrients you needed for a healthy pregnancy; now continue to make sure that you're replacing your reserves as they're used to create breastmilk.

 Alert

It's very important to make sure you get enough vitamin B-12. If you aren't eating any meat or dairy products, fortified nutritional yeast and some breakfast cereals are good sources; you may also want to consider a supplement either for yourself or your baby.

Most of the time, breastmilk is perfect even if the mother's diet isn't—the body will take what it needs, even if that means dipping into Mom's reserves. But some research suggests that if your diet is deficient in vitamin B-12, your milk will lack this essential vitamin, too.

For Both Vegetarians and Vegans

Both vegans and vegetarians should be careful to consume enough healthy fats. Choose soybean, olive, or canola oil for cooking. Some experts also recommend that vegetarians and vegans take a DHA supplement to ensure that they are getting enough essential fatty acids. Natural sources like flaxseed and walnuts do contain omega-3 fatty acids, but there is evidence that suggests that some people are unable to effectively convert those fats in their bodies.

Avoid artificial sweeteners. Try using natural sweeteners in small amounts, like honey, maple syrup, and juices. You can safely use stevia, a very sweet herb that is available in health-food stores and in many groceries.

Losing Weight Healthfully

The formula for weight loss is really pretty simple: to drop pounds, eat fewer calories and move your body more. But particularly during the postpartum months, it's very important that the calories you do eat are providing everything you need to recover and nourish yourself.

How Fast Will Weight Come Off?

When you give birth, you'll immediately drop around twenty pounds—anywhere from six to eight or more pounds for a healthy, full-term newborn, and another ten to fifteen or so when you consider your placenta and the fluids lost during and immediately after delivery. After that, you can expect to gain an extra pound or two when your milk comes in, but since you've still got some retained water to lose, and nursing burns, on average, 200 to 500 calories per day, you'll probably begin to drop more excess weight over the next few weeks. Most women lose the bulk in the first two weeks, and not much more from week two through six, though they notice a lot of changes in their bodies. At some point, that effortless weight loss will probably slow to a crawl, and you'll have to put in some extra effort to get back to your prepregnancy weight.

Don't Start Too Soon

Don't start the weight-loss process until your baby is at least two months old. In the first couple of months, you need to focus on healing your body, and that requires rest and good nutrition. If you're breastfeeding, it's even more important that you don't actively try to diet during this time. You need adequate nutrition to establish a good milk supply. Even if you aren't breastfeeding, you'll need as much energy as you can get to meet the demands of caring for a new baby, so eating enough good food is crucial to your health.

Take It Slow

You shouldn't lose more than 1 to 2 pounds per week, especially if you're breastfeeding. It's theorized that losing weight too quickly could release toxins from your body into your breastmilk, and rapidly dropping pounds can also affect your short- and long-term health, whether you're nursing or not.

And watch out for sudden drops in caloric intake—if you suddenly start eating a lot fewer calories, your milk supply, not to mention energy level, could suffer. Besides, suddenly eating less isn't an effective way to lose weight: your body will go into "starvation" mode, and your metabolism will slow down to hold on to the fat you've got.

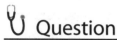 Question

Will breastfeeding make me lose weight faster?
Maybe. You'll burn extra calories simply by nursing, and many women find that fat just melts away while they're nursing. But some find that they have a harder time losing weight while nursing. This might be due to the body's desire to hold on to some extra padding for the future.

Even if you gained more weight than you would have liked during your pregnancy, don't rush yourself to take it off. A pound a week may not sound like fast enough weight loss to you, but that equals over twenty pounds in five months. Also, to lose just one pound a week, you need to burn off approximately 3,500 more calories than you take in—that's 500 calories a day, definitely enough to start with.

No Fads

Avoid fad diets in the postpartum months. Experts agree that the reason most fad diets work is that in eating a specific way, you restrict calories. But when you follow fad diets, you may restrict a lot more than just calories—you may be robbing yourself of necessary nutrients like enough fat, protein, or certain vitamins. And after people go off the fad diet, the weight comes back.

Chances are, you've heard of, or maybe tried, a fad diet or two in the past. And if you're hoping to drop a lot of pregnancy weight quickly, it might seem tempting to try one again. But remember that losing weight too quickly isn't good for you. Also, eliminating entire food groups from your diet is never a healthy way to eat, and is least healthy now that your body really needs good nutrition to heal well and give you the energy you need.

Another option is to try a modified version of the fad diet. For instance, say you tend to pig out on chips, cookies, and crackers and think going on a low-carb diet will help you lose weight. But the problem, in this case, isn't that you're eating carbs; it's that you're eating unhealthy, processed carbs full of sugar and sodium. Instead of shunning certain types of food, find healthy varieties of your favorites and eat them in moderation.

Essential

Some diet plans, like Weight Watchers, have created special plans for nursing mothers. As long as you're eating a balanced diet, consuming enough calories, and losing no more than 1 to 2 pounds per week, these plans are fine and may even give you the tools and accountability you need to eat a consistently healthy diet.

Tips for Postpartum Weight Loss

It isn't always easy to remember to eat well while you're adjusting to caring for a baby. You may forget to eat all morning, then binge on junk when your blood sugar plummets, or find yourself relying on fattening convenience and fast foods because you're too exhausted to prepare anything healthier. Here are some tips for eating well even when you're short on time, energy, and patience.

No Starvation

Don't let yourself get too hungry! If you forget to eat or wait too long between meals, your blood sugar can drop, leaving you irritable and shaky. And your body may go into the starvation mode we talked about earlier, meaning you won't be effectively burning calories anyway. Keep your energy level up and your metabolism buzzing along by eating smaller, balanced meals throughout the day.

Be Realistic

Studies show that most women can expect to take at least eight months to a year to return to their prepregnancy weight—and that's only if you gained no more than 30 pounds while pregnant. Whether you're breastfeeding or not, the year after you have a baby is a time of huge physiological change, which means your body is concentrating on more important things than dropping weight so you can squeeze back into your premommy jeans. If you focus more on eating to nourish your body and, in turn, your baby, you may be much more satisfied with the results of your "diet" than if you just count the numbers on the scale.

Eat Consciously

This can seem difficult to pull off if you're constantly juggling a baby under one arm, but one key to healthful eating is being aware of your hunger signals and paying close attention to what—and how much—food you're putting in your mouth.

Here are a few tips for eating consciously:

- Don't eat while standing up at the counter. Sit down at the table, and use a plate—and utensils.
- Don't eat while driving. Yes, going through a drive-thru can be a lifesaver when you've got a sleeping baby in the back seat, but at least stop the car while you eat your food. For one thing, driving and eating at the same time can be dangerous. For another, stuffing food in your face while you're paying

attention to the traffic around you makes it hard for you to really enjoy your food or recognize when you're full.

- Eat slowly, chewing each bite carefully before you swallow. Pay attention to the flavor, texture, and smell of your food. Resist the urge to shovel the food in. Your baby can snuggle in the sling or sit in a bouncy seat on the kitchen floor while you enjoy—instead of destroy—your meal.

- Don't talk on the phone or watch TV while you eat. Multitasking can only go so far, and one of the drawbacks is that it's very difficult to pay close attention to the task at hand. Most moms develop supreme multitasking skills when they've got babies, but save them for tasks that don't require your full attention, like folding laundry or loading the dishwasher.

- Eat only when you're hungry. When you get the urge to have a snack, pay attention to your motivation: are you truly feeling hunger pains, or is it something else? Stress, sadness, boredom, or low energy can all send you heading for the pantry when a nonfood fix would be a healthier solution.

- Lay off the soda and flavored soft drinks. That goes for diet and calorie-free beverages, too: recent research suggests that diet soda may actually trigger more calorie consumption. It's thought that the sweet flavor of artificially sweetened drinks isn't satisfying, but instead creates cravings for something else to gratify the drinker's sweet tooth. Regular sodas and other sweetened drinks are full of sugar and have little or no nutritive value. Stick to plain water, milk, or herbal tea.

- Make sure you're drinking enough water. Thirst can masquerade as hunger, and drinking enough water may help you feel fuller. Water with a squeeze of lemon or lime in it is a nice way to add some flavor without loading up with sugar.

Change Your Eating Outlook

If you're feeling deprived, it may be time for a different mindset when it comes to eating. Don't think of your eating habits in terms of dieting or restricting certain foods. Instead, try thinking about the foods you *must* eat every day, and start meals with those. Then, if you can't resist a snack afterward, you'll probably eat less of it—and it won't have taken the place of more healthy food.

Eat Balanced Meals

Eating protein with each meal will deliver longer-lasting energy. Many new moms skimp on protein in the morning, starting the day off with a sweet drink, sugary cereal, or pastry. Sugar-free yogurt—avoid the artificially-sweetened kind and go for the real stuff—cheese, and eggs will all give your breakfast more staying power and keep your blood sugar levels from crashing down midmorning.

Eat Healthfully on the Go

When you're eating on the go, be on the lookout for healthier alternatives to the usual burgers and fries. A baked potato, even with a dollop of sour cream or butter, is far healthier than fat-laden French fries. Many fast-food restaurants are beginning to offer surprisingly hearty salads; and as long as you don't drown them in fatty dressing, cheese, and bacon bits, they can be a healthy option. Also, when you're out of the house, take along baggies of your own favorite trail mix for a healthy treat.

Even with a perfect diet and exercise, you can expect your baby weight to take several months to melt away completely. In the meantime, the next chapter will help you choose a flattering transitional wardrobe that can help you feel pulled together and stylish while you're waiting to get back into your favorite prebaby clothes.

CHAPTER 14

Your Postpartum Wardrobe

WHEN YOU'RE A NEW MOM, there will be days when you feel saggy, tired, leaky, and just plain unattractive. A great-fitting pair of pants or a flattering shirt can give you a much-needed boost, but finding clothes that fit and flatter the postpartum body isn't always easy: huge, flowing clothes aren't usually flattering, and your prepregnancy wardrobe doesn't fit. But somewhere between your prepregnancy jeans and your stretch-panel maternity pants, there are clothes that will fit your new and still-changing shape.

The Early Weeks

Right after you've had your baby, you'll want to dress for comfort and function. Drawstring-waist pants and loose-fitting cotton tops are easy to nurse in and comfortable in the first days after giving birth.

Maternity Clothes

In the early weeks, many women just continue to wear maternity clothes. It can be depressing, but not as disheartening as continually trying to cram your new shape into ill-fitting prepregnant clothes. With maternity clothing getting more stylish and flattering every season, you probably have a lot of outfits that will look and fit great right now. Try on some of the clothing you were able to wear near the beginning of your pregnancy but grew out of; the fit may be trimmer than your end-of-pregnancy clothing while still providing enough room for comfort now.

Ⅼ⸌ Essential

Your husband's side of the closet may also be a great place to look for clothes. A man's button-down shirt or sweatshirt over a pair of leggings can make a comfy around-the-house outfit and will be easy to breastfeed in.

Transitional Pieces

Some maternity designers have also created transitional clothing—pieces like wraparound tops that can fit during or after pregnancy and are nursing friendly to boot. Also, many maternity clothes designers now make clothing that's intended for certain trimesters, like pants meant to be worn below the waist for the first and second trimesters, or shirts with a bit of extra room that aren't always long enough to make it to the end of a pregnancy. Pull out some of the clothes you discarded back around the fifth or sixth month of your pregnancy; they may fit great now.

Beyond Maternity Wear

As your middle continues to shrink, you lose more baby weight, and you start leaving the house, you'll probably want to get out of your PJs and maternity clothes and start wearing clothes that help you feel like you're getting back to normal.

Dressing for Your New Shape

Choosing a flattering wardrobe for the weeks and months after giving birth can be tricky. First of all, your body will probably not only be heavier, but also shaped differently than it was before you were pregnant. You may find extra fat clinging to your body in places you wouldn't have even considered before, like your inner thighs and upper back. If you had a boyish figure, your hips probably widened—

perhaps permanently—during pregnancy. You probably have some loose skin on your belly, and your abdomen might pooch out a little or a lot. Your breasts are probably significantly larger than they were before you were pregnant, especially if you're nursing.

With all those changes—and the knowledge that your body will continue to change over the months to come—try to choose clothing that will be well-fitting and flattering today, tomorrow, and next week.

Fabrics

When you're trying to create a wardrobe that's both figure flattering and easy to care for, you want to look for a few specific traits:

- **Wash-and-wear:** Who wants to worry about ironing, starching, hand washing, or dry cleaning? You've got better things to do, like kissing your baby's little fingers and toes. Pick clothes that can be thrown in the washing machine with the rest of your stuff. It's better yet if the fabric will resist wrinkles, especially if you occasionally leave clothes in the dryer overnight.
- **Nonclingy and matte:** Choose sturdy fabrics that skim over your curves without clinging. If you choose a jersey or other knit, look for a matte finish—shinier fabrics can highlight lumps and bumps.

Draw eyes Away from Your Tummy

If you're trying to downplay a larger middle, try wearing tops that draw the eye away from your center and bring them up toward your chest or neck. A detailed or interesting neckline, or chunky, eye-catching jewelry can do the trick.

Also remember to play up your assets. If you aren't crazy about your softer waistline but are in love with your more voluptuous breasts, try something that shows them off. A plunging neckline or scoop-neck top will show off your cleavage, while a high neck or halter top will accentuate the size of your new bust.

Use Color Wisely

Wear a dark color over the area you want to conceal and a brighter color on an area you'd like to accentuate. Tops that have a darker color over your belly and a brighter color near your face, or brightly colored or patterned sleeves can be very flattering and draw attention up and out, away from your middle.

For slimming and de-emphasizing bulges and bumps, black is a postpartum woman's friend. But remember that dark colors will show spit-up, so you may want to go with slimming colors with white patches or less-flattering light patterns that hide the spit-up.

Find a Forgiving Cut

If your belly still has some extra padding, stay away from snug, short tops. Loose peasant tops, dropped-waist styles that skim over your belly and end around your hips, flowing and asymmetrical hemlines, empire-waist styles, and shirts that camouflage your belly with strategically placed wraps, gathers, or tucks are all fashionable ways to conceal your still-shrinking tummy.

But What about Pants?

What's the skinny on low riders? It depends. Some moms like the way hip-hugging jeans don't press the flesh around the belly, which can cause unsightly squishing. Others find that low-waisted pants give them an unappealing "muffin top," where the excess stomach hangs over the waistband for all the world to see. On the other hand, high-waisted pants can feel like they're squashing your extra flesh and are often unflattering, drawing attention to the area of your body you'd most like to hide at this point. The trick seems to be in finding middle-of-the-road jeans that fit loosely enough to avoid tummy squashing, but are snug enough to pull in the looser skin on your lower abdomen and avoid that poochy, still-pregnant look. A lot will also depend on how the pants fit the rest of your shape, so you'll want to try on a few styles until you find one you like. Choose pants with a forgiving fit—you don't want to be bending over to pick up your baby and bust a seam—and if possible, a little stretch.

Dressing for Work

If you'll be heading back to work in the first six months to a year postpartum, chances are good that you'll be carrying some extra weight, especially around your middle, to the office with you. But don't be discouraged. Though you may not have your old figure back yet, you can still look sophisticated and stylish at work.

Follow these tips for choosing appropriate and figure-conscious office wear:

- Avoid pleated pants. Flat-front pants are the most flattering style for postpartum bellies.
- Wear jackets and blazers that nip in at the middle to create a waistline.
- Try tailored, fitted button-up shirts. They can be flattering and define your waist as long as they are made of a sturdy fabric that won't show every bulge, and don't fit too tightly.
- Don't spend a ton of money on a work wardrobe that you'll have to replace in a few months. To make the most of a few items, stick to black and neutral pieces, or buy pants and skirts in black and neutrals, saving colors for your tops. That way you'll be able to throw almost any two pieces together and make them work, which will give your wardrobe more mileage.
- Go for great accessories like shoes, handbags, scarves, and jewelry. These can give you and your wardrobe a pick-me-up, and you won't have to buy a new size later.
- Try trousers with vertical stripes for a slimming look. Wide-leg pants may also help balance out your middle.

Trying to squeeze into your prepregnancy work wear too soon will only leave you feeling awkward and uncomfortable, and this is not how you want to feel in a professional setting. Wearing clothes that fit your body and accentuate the parts you like will boost your self-esteem as you slowly slim down and regain your old shape.

Minimizing a Large Bust

Not every new mom celebrates the fullness of her new figure. If you're very large breasted, you may have a harder time finding flattering styles. You may find that the slits in nursing clothes aren't big enough or placed right to accommodate your breasts. You may also have a hard time finding nursing bras in your size. Here are some tips for dressing when you have very large breasts:

- V-neck and wrap-style shirts are flattering on larger bustlines. Try wearing dark colors on top, or choosing tops with a dark area in the chest to draw less attention to that part of your body.
- Look for tops or jackets with embellishments or gathers at the hips to draw attention away from your chest.
- Layers, like a wrap top over a tank, or a hoodie over a T-shirt, can help keep the emphasis off your bust.
- Check specialty lingerie shops, Web sites, and catalogs for nursing bras in your size. If you can't find nursing bras you like in your size, you can create your own by cutting around the top of a cup in a regular bra and stitching on clasps by machine or hand. You can buy special nursing-bra clasps on the Internet, but regular metal (plastic may break) swimsuit hooks, available in craft and sewing stores, work as well. If you aren't sure where to place the hooks, look at a nursing bra at a department store and copy the style. Or search online for instructions for making your own nursing bra.

Moms with large breasts often complain that regular nursing shirts don't work for them. You can try cutting holes or slits in a regular tank top, then layer it underneath a regular T-shirt. Or, if you're handy with a sewing machine, try making your own nursing tops. Buy two tank tops of a similar shape, fabric, and color. Cut the bottom third or so off of one, and the bottom three quarters or so off of the other. Keep the larger upper half with straps and the larger bottom half without straps. Hem the edges, slide the bottom piece into the top piece so that they overlap by a few inches, and sew them together, one seam horizontally across the back and two seams vertically on the sides. Now you'll have what looks like a single top with a large opening in the middle. To nurse, simply lift the upper portion—your breast will remain partially covered by the material of the tank top, and the bottom half of the outfit will cover your stomach. You can do this without a sewing machine if the top is made of a material that doesn't fray when it's cut.

Nursing Wear

Some women run out and buy an entire nursing wardrobe, while others make do with the clothing they've already got. But you don't need to break the bank with a whole new closet of clothes made specifically for breastfeeding. Try these tips for creating a nursing-friendly wardrobe with a few new pieces and the stuff you probably already have lying around.

The Layered Look

Pair a nursing camisole or tank top with a button-down shirt, cardigan sweater, jacket, tie-front top, or shrug sweater. You can buy a selection of inexpensive nursing tanks or camis in different colors and just rotate the sweaters and shirts you've already got over them. The nursing cami will make it easy to breastfeed discreetly, and you can wear some of your prepregnancy tops with them, even if you can't button them all the way anymore.

Full Coverage

When it comes to nursing-friendly clothing, think easy access and coverage. Many moms report that it's not the fear of accidentally flashing a bit of nipple that makes them reluctant to nurse in public, but the prospect of showing the world their stomachs. Also, exposing your belly on a chilly day can be really uncomfortable. Shirts that are large and loose have enough material to keep your stomach covered while you're nursing.

Shirts with Buttons

If you wear a button-down shirt without a tank or camisole under-neath it, you can either unbutton from the top down and pull your breast out the top, or unbutton from the bottom up. If you unbutton from the bottom up, it's easier to keep your breast from showing, but you may flash some tummy skin. If you button from the top down, you will eventually become good at keeping a hand over your breast until the baby's head blocks it from view.

Dressing Up

If you think you'll be attending any dress-up events with a nurs-ing baby (or if you'll need to pump breastmilk while dressed up), it's worthwhile to spend some of your nursing wardrobe budget on at least one breastfeeding-friendly dress. Many dresses are impossible to nurse or pump in without lifting the whole thing over your head, or unzipping it and taking the top down completely. A classic little black dress with nursing slits can be dressed up or down depend-ing on the occasion, and layered with a wrap or cardigan for colder weather.

Do It Yourself

Some moms make their own nursing-friendly tops by cutting slits in camisoles or tank tops, then wearing something over the top of them. When it's time to nurse you can lift one layer and pull your breast through the slit. The bottom tank will keep you mostly cov-ered up.

Give Nursing Clothes a Chance

Nursing wear is not what it used to be. Forward-thinking design-ers of maternity and nursing clothes are creating attractive, versatile styles you might not want to part with once you're done breastfeed-ing. While you can make do without nursing clothing if you shop carefully, select nursing-friendly tops from your current wardrobe, and maybe even take a pair of scissors to some nonbreastfeeding clothes, it's probably worth it to own a few fabulous nursing tops from a great designer, especially since the overall cut is likely to be flattering for your new-mom shape.

Selecting a Bra

Chances are you bought a few nursing bras during your pregnancy if you knew you'd be breastfeeding. But depending on how much your breasts change during the first weeks postpartum, you may find that the size you got doesn't work anymore, or you may discover that the style you chose doesn't offer enough support, isn't easy to open, or isn't as comfortable as you would have liked.

How Many Will You Need?

It's important to wear a clean nursing bra each day, since milk that leaks into your bra can breed fungus or bacteria. And some days you may experience a big leak that forces you to change bras again midday. Unless you feel like doing the laundry constantly, you'll probably want to have four or five bras on hand so that one is always sure to be clean.

If you find a nursing bra you absolutely love, it's probably a good idea to buy several of them, perhaps in different colors. Remember that bras look best under light-colored or sheer shirts when they're as close as possible to your own skin tone.

Stylish—and Even Sexy

Maybe you didn't buy any nursing bras at all. If the idea of a nursing bra conjures up the image of an industrial-strength white cotton over-the-shoulder boulder holder, think again. Nursing bras now come in a variety of colors, materials, shapes, fits, and styles. Styles include shelf-style bras built into camisoles, racerback styles, soft cup and underwire styles, crossover/wrap styles, and bras that open from the sides, middle, and top of the cups. They come in satin, cotton, polyester, and lace, and include padded cups. If you look beyond your discount department store, you'll find nursing bras in nude, black, and bright colors in addition to the traditional white.

Is Underwire Okay?

Underwire nursing bras create some controversy. Some moms feel that they provide the best shaping and support, but lactation experts agree that they can put pressure on your breasts, causing clogged ducts, which can lead to breast infections. At least in the beginning while you're establishing breastfeeding, it's best to avoid underwire bras unless you can't get comfortable support with any other style. Later, when your milk supply has evened out and you know whether you're prone to clogged ducts or not, you can decide whether wearing an underwire is a risk worth taking for you.

 Alert

Not all underwire bras are built the same way. When you're trying on an underwire bra, take note of where the wire lies and how it looks and feels. It should lie flat against your skin without sticking out on the sides, and shouldn't chafe, rub, or pinch your breast or armpit tissue.

Fabric

Cotton is always a good choice for nursing bras. It's breathable, which can help your nipples stay dry and healthy. Make sure the cotton is prewashed, so you don't end up with a shrunken bra after a few washes. Sometimes, 100-percent cotton bras don't provide enough support, or may become stretched out or loose. Polyester-cotton blends may hold their shape a little better, and sometimes may provide better support. If you're not prone to thrush and are diligent about changing your nursing pads and washing bras frequently, a polyester-cotton blend is probably fine. Lace cups are very breathable, but they won't do much to stop the flow of milk, and may not be quite as pretty if you can see your nursing pads through them. Make sure any lace isn't itchy or irritating to your skin.

Openings and Other Details

Nursing bras generally have one of three kinds of openings: hook and eye, plastic clasp, or snaps. Hook-and-eye closures usually offer several rows of eyes, offering an easily customizable fit. Snaps and plastic clasps may not be as adjustable, and if the bra gets stretched out or your breasts shrink, bras with this type of clasp may start to feel too loose or bunchy. Some nursing bras don't have any closures but can be pulled to the side or up to nurse. You can use this type of bra for sleeping in if it's not supportive enough for daytime use. Just make sure that when you pull it up or over, the material doesn't compress your breast at all. You may want to pick bras with different types of openings to wear with different outfits.

What's Your Size?

Bra sizes consist of a letter, or cup size, and a number, or band size. Bra manufacturers use a variety of formulas for coming up with these sizes, so for the best fit, you'll want to get measured by a professional bra fitter at a specialty lingerie shop or high-end department store, or follow detailed instructions in the manufacturer's catalog or at their Web site.

If possible, it's best to be fitted for a nursing bra in the last month of pregnancy. Nursing bras can usually handle the increased fullness you'll experience during engorgement and still fit after the engorgement goes away. On the other hand, if you try to get fitted for a bra while engorged, it'll be difficult to know just how much your breasts will shrink as the engorgement subsides, and the fit may not be as good.

Remember, your breast isn't just a number and a letter. It's also got its own unique shape, which may make certain styles work better for you, and some not work at all. One of your breasts may be bigger or shaped differently than the other, so bras that allow adjustment in the straps and band may help you get a better fit.

If You Aren't Nursing

If you aren't breastfeeding, chances are good your breasts still went through changes during pregnancy and you may not be able to wear your old bras again, or you may find they don't give your new breasts enough shape and support. Wait until any engorgement has gone away, and then shop for a new bra. Your breasts may go back to the size they were prepregnancy, stay a little larger, or even shrink. You might also find that they're saggier than they were before, so you may need to experiment with some different styles and fits until you find one that's comfortable and flattering.

Other Undergarments

Some specialty shops sell support garments specially meant to be worn in the postpartum weeks. These can be comfortable during the early weeks, when you feel like your organs are all shifting around, and can even reduce afterpain discomfort. They also have the added bonus of working as a sort of gentle girdle, keeping saggy tummy skin in place and smoothing your outline. Sometimes these garments look like a pair of high-waisted underwear, and sometimes they're more akin to a weight lifter's belt.

Nursing Wear for Nighttime

At night, you can choose from a variety of nursing gowns and pajamas, but be aware that it's not always easy to find the slits in the middle of the night. Sometimes, simply sleeping in a fitted T-shirt or tank is easiest, since you can simply pull it up and won't have to worry about any extra fabric. If you usually like to sleep in the nude, you may just want to wear a soft sleeping bra. It'll give you some support and prevent you from leaking all over the bed, without being too cumbersome or bulky.

If you think nursing will hinder your ability to surprise your partner by wearing sexy lingerie to bed, think again. A growing number of retailers, including specialty Web sites and catalogs, are now selling sexy nursing gowns and pajamas as well as matching nursing bra-and-panty sets in lace and satin, and in colors like racy red and black. Some even have matching nursing pads.

CHAPTER 15

Postpartum Depression and Other Postpartum Mood Disorders

WHILE POSTDELIVERY HORMONE fluctuations combined with loss of sleep, the psychological and physical adjustment to motherhood, and the reality that you've made a huge life change by giving birth can lead any mother to feel emotional, sometimes sadness, anger, or anxiety can go beyond the baby blues. In this chapter you'll learn about postpartum depression and anxiety, as well as lesser-known postpartum mood disorders like postpartum obsessive-compulsive disorder, postpartum psychosis, and postpartum panic disorder.

What Is a Postpartum Mood Disorder?

Many people confuse the baby blues with postpartum depression, or think that postpartum depression is the only psychiatric condition related to the postpartum period. The baby blues occur in up to 80 percent of women and are characterized by weepiness, anxiety, difficulty focusing, and mood swings. You may find yourself switching from crying to laughing in a heartbeat or feel especially vulnerable or worried about the baby. The baby blues aren't considered a disorder. They're caused by the emotional highs and lows that go along with the experience of birth, sleep deprivation, stress, and the normal hormonal shifts of the postpartum period. If you've been suffering from the baby blues, your symptoms are likely to be less severe than full-blown depression, and they'll go away without treatment. Beyond the baby blues, there are five distinct postpartum mood disorders.

Postpartum Depression and Anxiety

Being temporarily sad, anxious, or unhappy is a normal part of being human and not necessarily a cause for concern. But if your feelings of sadness or worries interfere with your ability to enjoy your life or function from day to day, it can be signs of something more serious. When this happens in the weeks and months after giving birth, it's called postpartum depression or anxiety, and if untreated it can interfere with your ability to enjoy your new baby and the experience of motherhood.

Symptoms

Experts say that postpartum depression is extremely common and often goes unrecognized, masked by the normal fatigue, sleeping troubles, moodiness, and other changes that women naturally go through when they have young babies. Here is a list of symptoms that often indicate postpartum depression or anxiety:

- Sadness or hopelessness
- Anxiety or feeling very overwhelmed
- Restlessness or irritability
- Loss of appetite
- Emotional eating
- Unexplained or uncontrollable crying
- A lack of energy or motivation
- Sleeplessness
- Wanting to sleep all the time
- Loss of interest in the things that would usually bring you joy or fun
- Difficulty remembering things or focusing on a task
- Not wanting to be around family or friends
- Headaches, heart palpitations, or hyperventilation
- Being afraid you may hurt the baby
- Being afraid you may hurt yourself
- Taking no interest in the baby

Causes

Postpartum depression and anxiety can often be linked to stress caused by the challenges of new motherhood, anxiety over whether you'll be a good mother, lack of sleep or physical fatigue, or hormonal shifts. After you give birth, the amount of estrogen and progesterone in your body drops swiftly, sometimes triggering mood swings. And your thyroid gland, which helps to regulate your metabolism, may also slow down its output of hormones a few months after you give birth, leading to depression-like symptoms including sadness, a feeling of blah-ness, irritability, sleep problems, weight gain, difficulty concentrating, memory loss, and extreme tiredness.

Risk Factors

If you have a family history of depression, were depressed during pregnancy, had a stressful or traumatic birth or a sick or premature baby, or if you are socially isolated, you are at a higher risk of developing postpartum depression or anxiety.

Other Postpartum Mood Disorders

Unfortunately, postpartum depression isn't the only mood disorder to be watchful for after giving birth. There are a few other disorders that affect women postpartum, including postpartum obsessive-compulsive disorder, postpartum panic disorder, postpartum psychosis, and posttraumatic stress disorder. These disorders affect significantly fewer women compared to postpartum depression and anxiety, but you should still be aware of their signs and symptoms.

Postpartum Obsessive-Compulsive Disorder

PPOCD is more unusual than postpartum depression, occurring in between 3 and 5 percent of new mothers. A mother suffering from PPOCD may find herself having obsessive, sometimes violent thoughts about her baby. Or she may develop compulsive habits such as checking again and again to make sure the windows are locked or the stove is turned off. Sometimes PPOCD will manifest as an obsession with cleanliness. Sometimes a mother with PPOCD will have persistent and unwanted thoughts about hurting or killing her baby, which may horrify her. She may be afraid to be alone with the baby, even if she doesn't believe she would ever really act on the visions in her head.

If you or anyone in your family has a history of obsessive-compulsive behavior, you're at a greater risk of developing the condition during the postpartum period. Therapy and antidepressant medication can be helpful for treatment of PPOCD, as can connecting with other mothers who've experienced it.

Postpartum Panic Disorder

About 10 percent of postpartum women experience extreme anxiety and panic attacks. Often, these panic attacks can seem to come from nowhere, and they can be very frightening—people sometimes describe a panic attack as feeling like a heart attack.

Thyroid dysfunction and a family history of panic attacks may make you more inclined to develop postpartum panic disorder. If you think you might be suffering from postpartum panic disorder, see a doctor for treatment, who may recommend therapy or medication.

Postpartum Psychosis

Postpartum psychosis is an extreme form of postpartum depression. It's more common in women with certain pre-existing psychiatric problems, like bipolar disorder. Women suffering from postpartum psychosis may experience hallucinations, delusions, mania, and troubling or obsessive thoughts about the baby. Postpartum psychosis is rare, but it can be serious, as it has been linked to a high rate of suicide and infanticide. If you feel out of control, worry about harming yourself or your baby, or hear voices or see things that no one else can, you may be suffering from postpartum psychosis and should seek medical attention immediately. Treatment may include hospitalization and antipsychotic medications.

Posttraumatic Stress Disorder

If your birth was very difficult, ended in an unwanted c-section, resulted in injury to you, or if your baby was born early, became sick, or died, you could develop what's known as posttraumatic stress disorder (PTSD). Most people associate this condition with accident or trauma victims, or soldiers who experience flashbacks from war. But mental-health experts are beginning to realize that a traumatic birth experience can bring on the same sort of symptoms.

 Alert

> The death of a baby can be a huge trigger for postpartum depression and other mood disorders. If your baby died during or soon after birth, you may need special help working through your emotions afterward. See Chapter 19 for more information on postpartum care after a loss.

Women with this condition may experience flashbacks, intense anxiety, nervousness or jitters, insomnia, rage, disturbing dreams, or even hallucinations. Mothers with PTSD are, not surprisingly, also more likely to suffer from postpartum depression, though it's also thought that some cases of PPD may actually be misdiagnosed PTSD. If you can't stop having upsetting thoughts or dreams about your birth, if things that bring up memories of birth cause you a lot of distress, or if you ever have flashbacks or feel like you are reliving your birth experience, you may be suffering from postpartum PTSD.

Is It Your Thyroid?

If you're exhausted and sluggish, and are gaining weight or unable to lose weight, you may assume you're suffering from standard-issue postpartum depression. But as mentioned previously, postpartum hormone shifts can cause dysfunction of the thyroid gland, also known as postpartum thyroiditis. It's not known exactly how common postpartum thyroiditis is, but increasingly a sluggish or hyperactive thyroid gland is being recognized as a possible contributor to depressive symptoms and fatigue. It's also possible that postpartum thyroiditis is not diagnosed as often as it could be because it's mistaken for garden-variety sleep deprivation or baby blues.

Symptoms and Causes

If the thyroid is producing too many hormones, it can cause anxiety, weight loss, or insomnia. If it's producing too few, it can cause weight gain and fatigue. Often, your thyroid goes through a cycle of overproduction in the first few months postpartum, followed by underproduction after the third month.

Diagnosis and Treatment

If you are experiencing these symptoms and think it could be related to your thyroid, it can't hurt to have a blood test to check your thyroid levels. Other symptoms of postpartum thyroiditis may include dry skin, intolerance to cold, muscle weakness, constipation, and goiter, which is when the thyroid gland in your neck becomes swollen.

Often, postpartum thyroiditis resolves on its own, but thyroid hormone replacement therapy or beta-blocking medication are possible treatments. If anyone in your family suffers from thyroid disease or if you have insulin-dependent diabetes, you are at a higher risk of developing postpartum thyroiditis.

Preventing Depression

There's not a whole lot you can do about the hormonal shifts that come with the postpartum period. Your body is adjusting itself and working to return to its prepregnancy state, which can mean discomfort and emotional distress for you. While these effects are somewhat inevitable, there are measures you can take to prevent these hormone changes from developing into full-blown postpartum depression.

Rest Up

Not getting enough sleep is a major factor in postpartum depression. Do whatever you have to do to get more rest. Lack of adequate sleep can alter your brain chemistry, and fatigue can make even the most everyday tasks seem insurmountable. Nap when your baby naps, get somebody to come hold the baby for you so you can get some extra sleep, and ask your partner to take over the last hour or so of the evening so you can go to bed early.

Go Easy on Yourself

If you're putting too much pressure on yourself to keep a perfect house or be a perfect mother, a sense of failure will almost always follow—nobody's perfect! Relax your standards when it comes to non-essentials. It's okay if your house gets a little messy while your baby is little. If living in clutter just adds to your feelings of stress and anxiety, consider hiring help—a professional organizer or a housekeeper—to come help you get things in order.

Get Connected

Being socially isolated is a recipe for depression. Moms need other adult company, and sympathetic ears to listen and commiserate. The Internet has made it possible to make connections with other mothers all across the country, which can be helpful, but a computer friendship can only go so far—it's important to go beyond your monitor. Instead of spending all your time socializing on parenting message boards, try using the Internet as a way to hook up with moms in your own community, and meet up in real life. This will give you a good reason to get out of your pajamas and see some sunlight.

See the Light

Seasonal affective disorder, or SAD, is a depressive disorder that usually happens in the late fall and early winter and is connected to a lack of sunlight. It affects between 10 and 20 percent of the American population, most of them women in their twenties, thirties, and forties. Though SAD isn't specifically linked to the postpartum period, women who are already prone to suffering from SAD may find that being inside most of the time with a new baby can bring on symptoms, and SAD on top of postpartum depression can exacerbate the symptoms. If you live in a colder climate, you're more likely to suffer from SAD. Spending some time outside every day during peak sun hours (between noon and 2 P.M. if possible) can help.

Move Your Body

Energy breeds energy. Exercise is linked to a lower incidence of postpartum depression, and no wonder: not only does it produce feel-good endorphins, but it can increase your energy level and endurance, help you look better and feel healthier, and get you out in the fresh air and sun on a regular basis. If you can't imagine where you'll find the energy to exercise, start small. Lace up your shoes, put your baby in a stroller, and go for a stroll around the block. For extra motivation, get a friend to stop by every day and take you out with her. You may find that expending a little energy actually gives you back even more.

Ľ. Essential

Full-spectrum light bulbs, which mimic natural lighting and can be used as overhead lights or in lamps, and therapeutic light boxes can be helpful in easing the symptoms of SAD. You can purchase these products at ✑www.sadlight.com.

Give Nutrition a Boost

If your diet is lacking, you may be robbing your body and brain of the foods you need to keep your energy levels up and regulate your moods. For instance, diets deficient in DHA (docosahexaenoic acid), found in healthy fats like fish oil and soy and canola oils, and B vitamins, found in dark green leafy vegetables, eggs, meat, and dairy products, have been linked to a higher incidence of depression.

To protect yourself against diet-induced depression, keep taking your prenatal vitamin while you're breastfeeding, and be sure to eat a healthy, balanced diet containing whole, unprocessed grains; fruits and veggies; and healthy fats.

 Alert

> Certain herbal products are credited with reducing depression. But it's important to keep in mind that herbs can be strong medicines and must be used with respect, especially if you're nursing or taking other medications at the same time. Check with an experienced herbalist or naturopath before you start an herbal regimen.

Help Others

If you're bored and feeling blah, it may help to get out into your community and take on a volunteer project or other activity that interests you and sparks your passion. Helping others is a great way to take your mind off your own troubles and has the built-in benefit of connecting you with other people, which can help prevent depression.

Give Yourself Direction

Even if you shun schedules, a flexible routine can help keep you moving through your day and help you avoid that aimless feeling that can be, well, depressing. Babies usually thrive on flexible routines, and eventually your baby's sleeping and eating schedule may even out if you provide a predictable pattern to the day. If you know roughly what to expect from your day, you may find you have an easier time getting things done and feeling a sense of accomplishment and order.

Banish Guilt

Guilt is a downward spiral: you feel guilty because you aren't a "good-enough" mother, wife, homemaker, friend, employee . . . well, you get the picture. And then, you spend so much time feeling guilty that you withdraw from life, and feel even worse about yourself. Remind yourself that nobody is perfect. Don't spend time with people who make you feel bad about yourself or your parenting style or skills. Find friends who give you a boost.

Essential

Starting the morning off too slowly can make it hard to get moving later. You may want to get up with your spouse in the morning and plan some errands, a walk, or a Mommy and Me class first thing to start off the day with action instead of inertia.

Shun Stress

Avoid stressful events like moving or taking a new, more taxing job during the postpartum period if you can. Major life changes can add stress, which can lead to depression or anxiety. If watching the news makes you anxious, turn it off—permanently. If interactions with specific people always leave you stressed out to the point that you can't stop thinking about it, keep your distance for a while.

Try to Look at the Bright Side

Dwelling on the dark side is no way to improve your mood. It's normal to feel sadness and anxiety sometimes, but try to balance it with laughter and a sense of perspective. If you naturally lean toward the gloomy or pessimistic side, you might have to give yourself a nudge. Try making a list of things you are grateful for: a warm bed, your partner, your baby, friends and family, your daily cup of coffee. Also, make a concerted effort to find something to laugh at each day, whether it's a sitcom you love or the comments of a hilarious friend. It may feel forced at first to try to work happy moments into your life, but they really can add up to a better outlook overall.

Treating Depression and Anxiety

Sometimes even if you do everything in your power to stay cheerful and focus on the joy of your new baby, postpartum depression can take hold. This doesn't mean you've done anything wrong or are an unfit mother; hormonal changes are beyond your control. Luckily, there are several treatment options available to you if you feel like you're suffering from postpartum depression.

Talk Therapy

Sometimes, talking through your worries and concerns with a third party like a counselor or psychologist can help you cope with your feelings. If your depression is mild, therapy, combined with the lifestyle changes described above, may be enough to make you feel better.

Medication

If your depression is more severe, talking it through may not be enough. There are several antidepressant medications that are considered safe for nursing babies, including Zoloft and Paxil. Experts agree that, while some antidepressants may pose a small risk to the baby, the risks of untreated postpartum depression are more serious. You may also want to consult with a good naturopath or homeopath for effective alternative treatments.

If you worry that some of the medication may pass through to your breastmilk, keep in mind that if you're unable to interact with or enjoy your baby it can have a negative effect on her development. Talk with your care provider and carefully weigh the medication's possible risks and benefits.

If your depression is mild, your care provider may recommend that you start with talk therapy or make some other changes in your life before you opt for medication. Also, keep in mind that most studies show that negative effects of certain antidepressants on a nursing baby happen in the first couple of months postpartum. If your baby is older than that, his chances of side effects are far less.

L. Essential

Not all doctors are knowledgeable about antidepressants and breastfeeding, so it's a good idea to arm yourself with information before you see a doctor. A good resource for finding out more about the possible effects a drug might have on your milk and your baby is *www.ibreastfeeding.com.*

Do You Really Need to Seek Treatment?

If you aren't happy, it can affect everything about motherhood, from the bond you share with your baby to the care you're able to give her and older children, if you have them, to the memories you'll have later. Untreated depression in mothers can have a huge negative effect on children all the way through adolescence and is linked to language and developmental delays, behavior problems, trouble making and keeping friends, and problems in school. Depression can also have a negative effect on your marriage and other relationships. And depression during your baby's early months can keep you from enjoying the experience of motherhood. Don't allow yourself to feel like a failure or less of a mother because you need to seek treatment for postpartum depression. It's crucial that you seek help so that you can fully participate in your baby's life, now and as he grows.

While mild depression may be something you can overcome yourself with changes to your lifestyle, more serious depression and mood disorders should not be ignored. If you aren't feeling like yourself or can't find joy in your new baby, it's worth it to make a call to your care provider and see what's going on. Depression, anxiety, and other mood disorders can rob you of your energy, optimism, joy, and self-esteem, and make it difficult for you to be an engaged, happy, and confident mother. You owe it both to yourself and your baby to feel as good as you can both physically and emotionally.

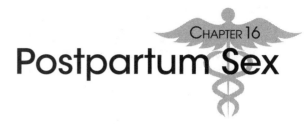

Chapter 16

Postpartum Sex

AT SOME POINT AFTER giving birth, you (or your partner) will probably start thinking about resuming your prebaby sex life. There are a number of issues that can complicate postpartum sex, so it's important for both you and your partner to be patient and accepting of your healing, your new body, and your changed priorities now that you are parents. This chapter covers important considerations for postpartum sex, from your emotions to birth control.

Are You Physically Ready?

When it comes to resuming sex after giving birth, you've probably heard the six-week guideline. But that's just a rough estimate of when it might be okay for you to start having sex again. Some women may be ready earlier, and many women may need more time.

Bleeding

Generally, it's considered safe to start having sex again once your postpartum bleeding, or lochia, has stopped. This indicates that your uterus has healed and sex is no longer considered an infection risk. If you're still bleeding, it could mean that your cervix is still open, leaving your uterus vulnerable to bacteria.

Some women have stop-and-start lochia after a few weeks. If you stop bleeding at a few weeks postpartum, it doesn't necessarily mean that you've healed completely or that sex is a good idea. Check with your care provider to be sure.

Your Bottom

You'll also want to take your perineal area into consideration. If you had stitches, tearing, or an episiotomy, your perineum may be tender for weeks. Deep tears will take longer to heal than surface tears and you may need more time than the standard six weeks of healing. Even if your perineum or vaginal tissue doesn't feel sore during normal activity, sexual intercourse may be too uncomfortable or even painful to be enjoyable in the first couple of months. If you had a cesarean section, you'll need to make sure your incision is healing properly—no tenderness, oozing, or redness—before starting to have sex again, even if you've passed the six-week mark. If you aren't sure, ask your care provider.

Emotional Concerns

Even if you've gotten the green light and feel physically ready for sex, you'll probably still have some questions and concerns. Even if your body has healed enough to begin again, you may not feel emotionally ready. The following sections cover some common concerns you and your partner may experience.

Your Partner

It's very common for your partner to be nervous the first time you have sex after your baby is born. He may be worried about hurting you. He may be unsure of himself and also uncertain of his role in your life now that you're devoting so much time and attention to your baby.

Also, watching you give birth may have temporarily changed the way your husband feels about you sexually. While many men report feeling even more loving and attracted to their wives after watching them give birth and nurse babies, some men may have a harder time coping with their partners' new role and changes to her body. This is normal and should pass with time.

You

While it's possible your partner might not feel ready for sex at the six-week mark, it could also be the other way around: your partner is all over you, wanting sex to resume as quickly as possible, and you just don't feel ready. You might be worried that sex will hurt, that you'll get pregnant again soon, that your partner won't be turned on by your new body, or that your baby will wake up in the middle and interrupt you. Remember, the first few times having sex postpartum don't have to be perfect, and with time and patience, the issues that worry you can be resolved. You will grow more comfortable in your changed body, your perineum will heal, and sex will become more and more comfortable and enjoyable.

 ## Alert

Even if you haven't had a period yet, as mentioned in Chapter 11, you may still be fertile. It's very important to address the family-planning issue before you start having sex again, even though it may feel strange after nine months of being able to have sex without worrying about pregnancy. Your midwife or doctor will probably speak with you about birth-control options at your six-week checkup. Revisit Chapter 11 for more information on birth control and family-planning options.

As for being interrupted, parents of young children soon come to expect and accept interruptions as just another part of the deal. Accept that your sex life will be different, and that you and your partner can find creative ways to meet both your needs for intimacy and sex within your new roles as parents.

Comfort Issues

Even if you feel completely healed most of the time, sex can remind you quickly that you've recently given birth. You may feel sore, tight, or uncomfortable during intercourse. This doesn't mean you have to put off sex, but you may need to make some adjustments to make you feel more comfortable. Using lubricant and experimenting with different positions could be a big help.

Use a Lubricant

Vaginal dryness, which often goes hand in hand with breastfeeding, can make sex much more uncomfortable than it needs to be. This dryness may seem even more evident if you're using condoms for birth control, as the latex can rub against sensitive tissues and cause friction. Using a lubricant can help. However, as mentioned previously, if you're using latex condoms or a rubber or latex diaphragm or cervical cap, you cannot use an oil-based lubricant like petroleum jelly, hand lotion, or baby oil, since oils break down latex. Instead, use plenty of a water-based lubricant like KY jelly, liquid, or mist, and go slowly. Plenty of foreplay may help, especially if you can have an orgasm before you begin intercourse.

Experiment with Positions

You can expect some discomfort the first few times you have sex, but if it really hurts or is very uncomfortable, stop and try something new. One thing that can make a big difference is the positions you use.

During pregnancy, you probably had to get creative with sexual positions as your belly grew. Now, the positions that were your favorites then may not feel quite as good. Depending on your body and where you're feeling pain or discomfort, changing position—say, from missionary to lying on your side with your partner behind you—may help take pressure or friction off of a sore area.

Some women like being on top because it gives them more control over penetration and speed. Experiment until you find something that works for both of you, and don't forget to add more lubricant whenever things start to feel stuck or the friction becomes too intense.

Lack of Desire

When you're caring for a new baby all day and much of the night, chances are good that there will be times you'd rather sleep, take a bath, or do pretty much anything other than have sex. There are a few reasons for this reduced sex drive:

- You may be sleep deprived, which can make sex sound exhausting rather than fun. Not to mention, it might cut into available nap time.
- The hormonal changes that come with suppressed ovulation, postpartum fluctuations, and nursing can also cause a low libido.
- Many women simply feel "touched-out" by the end of a day of snuggling and caring for a new baby, and don't particularly want that much physical contact with another person.
- It's also been suggested that lower sexual desire is nature's way of making sure new moms don't get pregnant again too quickly.
- You may feel frustrated by the time constraints that having a baby in the house may put on your sex life.

Whatever the reasons, while motherhood doesn't make you a less sexual being, it can temporarily dampen your desires. By accepting that your sex life will probably be different than it was prebaby and coming up with creative ways to stay intimate, you and your partner can make sure both your needs are met.

Keep It Short

If you don't feel like you'll have the energy for a lengthy sexual encounter, be honest with your partner. He may feel like he has to perform by having sex for hours, when you'd prefer a shorter session. Chances are your partner would gladly choose a passionate quickie over no sex at all. Don't worry that he'll be offended if you'd rather not make it an all-nighter. Just be honest—tell him that you would like to have sex, but are also very tired and don't know if you have the energy for a long session. If you keep the lines of communication open, you can find a way to meet both your needs without either partner feeling shoved aside or pressured.

Accept the Changes

You and your husband or partner may have to adjust your expectations about how often you'll be having sex when your baby is very young. Don't feel like you have to match the intensity of your prebaby love life or meet some arbitrary goal for how much sex you should be having. Less-frequent sex is only a problem if one of you is dissatisfied with how much you're getting. If you're hoping for sex once a month while he was thinking five times a week would be great, you may have to do some compromising.

Keep Communicating

For many men, physical closeness is essential to feeling loved. You'll want to be sure your husband or partner doesn't feel like the baby has replaced him in your life, and find ways to help meet his needs. On the other hand, it's important for your partner to understand where you're coming from and not pressure you into sex before you're ready or expect you to be willing whenever he's in the mood.

Essential

If your partner's sexual expectations of you are more than you feel up to filling, sit down and have a talk with him. Make sure he understands that it's not that you don't find him attractive or that you love the baby more, but that you're tired and having a hard time getting in the mood to have sex right now.

You may want to stress that the easier he can make things for you around the house, the more likely that you'll have the energy and be in the frame of mind for sex. You don't want sex to turn into a bargaining chip—"I've done the dishes, now you're obligated to get busy!"—but it can be useful for your husband to understand that not getting sleep, caring for a baby 24/7, and doing housework all sap your energy.

Your partner may find that the more he pitches in directly correlates to how much desire you can muster up when the time comes. For more information on communicating with your partner about sex, intimacy, housework, and more, see Chapter 18.

Make Time for You

It's also very important that you get regular time alone to recharge your batteries. It's unreasonable for you to expect yourself to be on call 24/7 as a mother, and also find the mental and physical energy for feeling sexy. For many women it takes stepping out of one role for a moment before they can step into the other.

L. Essential

Sex toys like vibrators can add a level of newness and excitement during a time when you may need to kick things up a notch to locate your libido. They can also be an efficient way to get you in the mood or bring you to orgasm quickly if you're short on time before the baby wakes up.

Give Yourself Prep Time

Since so much of a woman's experience of sex is in her head, it's very possible to go from 0 to 60 if you put yourself in the right frame of mind. If you have a hard time getting in the mood, let your partner put the baby to sleep while you take a bath or enjoy a glass of wine. Some women find that erotic material like books, magazine stories, or movies bring them out of their "mommy mind" and bring out the sexual side that's snoozing beneath the surface.

Let Him Convince You

Some women find that, even if they don't feel like having sex initially, a little convincing can sometimes get them in the mood. But that shouldn't translate into pressure for you. Let your husband know that you enjoy spending time kissing and being together, and that it may or may not lead to sex down the road. Either way, you'll have gotten the benefit of being physically close. If you still really aren't in the mood to make love, maybe you can find another way to satisfy your partner through oral sex or mutual masturbation. It's not necessarily the intercourse that's important here—it's showing affection and expressing love through physical intimacy that can be so important to both you and your partner, and you may be able to find a variety of ways to satisfy him sexually even when you aren't up for intercourse. If you just don't have the energy for sex or don't find it pleasurable yet, think of other ways to express the intimacy that can keep you close as lovers now that you are also co-parents.

Take Charge

Don't always wait for your husband or partner to initiate. If you feel like he's coming to you for sex all the time and you're always putting him off or pushing him away, he may soon begin to feel ignored, and you may feel put-upon—especially if he tends to want to have sex at the same time that you're thinking about sleep. Instead, find a time of day when you have more energy, and surprise him by initiating romance. You may find that you're more in the mood when you thought of it first, and he won't have to feel like he's always bugging you for sex.

When He's Not in the Mood

Some women find that their husbands don't want to have sex as much as they do when the baby is small. Not all men want to have sex all the time—your partner may be just as tired as you are, or he may be anxious about caring for a baby or providing for his family, making it hard for him to think about sex. If your husband doesn't want to be intimate with you at all, talk to him about it and see if you can get to the root of the problem.

Alert

> While fluctuations in libido can be normal, a complete lack of sex drive in a man could indicate a physical or emotional issue that you might need to address, especially if he once had a high sex drive and things changed suddenly.

Better Than Before

Some women find that their sex life improves after having a baby. For some women, the process of pregnancy and birth empowers them and helps them feel more in touch with their sensual and sexual side. Others find that the changes to their bodies make sex more enjoyable or that they are better able to have orgasms. If you aren't having a great time with sex right away, remember that your body is still going through many changes. You may find that a few months or a year down the road, your sex life will be better than ever.

Finding the Time—and Place—for Romance

Now that there is this new baby in your life—and possibly right there in your bedroom with you—you're probably finding it more difficult to create a romantic atmosphere with your partner. This isn't necessarily a bad thing, though. You may just have to get creative when it comes to the time and place for sex.

Plan for Spontaneity

As your baby gets older, he'll begin sleeping for longer stretches at night and taking more regular naps, so you can plan for romantic interludes. But in the early months, your sex life may be catch-as-catch-can. Rethink the idea that there's a "right" time or place for sex, and take this opportunity to be spontaneous and a bit wild. A quickie in the bathroom or walk-in closet can be a fun adventure that you can fit in while your baby is sleeping.

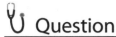

Question

Will my baby be traumatized if she wakes up while my husband and I are having sex?
It can be a mood killer to look over during sex and realize that your baby is awake and watching you, but she has no concept of what you're doing. Don't worry—you won't cause her emotional damage.

Employ a Sitter

Ask a grandparent, godparent, aunt, or uncle if he or she would like to take your baby on an errand, and use that time for a quick romp. When your baby is big enough and you're comfortable being away from her for a few hours, you can plan for a romantic date night complete with dinner *and* dessert.

Keep It Light

You can also try re-creating a romantic date at home after your baby's gone to bed. Just remember that seduction and sex aren't going to go perfectly every time. Sometimes, the baby will wake up crying, which can lead to laughter or frustration. You'll have to decide whether to keep going with crying or cooing in the background—not always the best way to keep the mood going—or try again later. Knowing ahead of time that you may be interrupted can help keep you from setting your expectations too high and ending up frustrated.

Being Intimate Without Having Sex

There's no way around it: In those first weeks and months after the baby is born, there will be times when you or your partner just won't want to have sex. You'll both have a lot on your minds—not to mention your busy schedules—and by the time the sun goes down, you'll often be hoping for a nice deep sleep rather than a romantic encounter.

But while you may prefer to use your bed only for sleep some days, it's very important to keep intimacy and romance alive during these months. Even when your libido is low, intimate moments between you will help ensure that both you and your partner feel valued and loved. Kissing and hugging often, giving shoulder rubs and back massages, eating dinner together by candlelight with romantic music in the background, or taking a bath or shower together are ways you can reconnect and be intimate with your husband, even if it doesn't always lead to sex. But you may also find that these romantic gestures lead to you feeling sexy more often than you had anticipated.

Adjusting to Motherhood

THE POSTPARTUM PERIOD is more than just physically taxing; it can also be a time when you feel vulnerable, emotional, and unsure of your competence as a mother and just what your new role means. From dealing with the myths and realities of motherhood to trying to hold on to your identity, to bonding with your baby and getting through the day without feeling like you've accomplished absolutely nothing, adjusting to the role of Mom can be a challenge.

Motherhood: Myths and Realities

You've probably read a book or magazine article that started with something like "you may be feeling ambivalent about pregnancy" and ended with "But don't worry, as soon as you're holding that baby in your arms, you'll know you were always meant to be a mother."

As nice as it would be to believe that this is always true, real life doesn't always include a fairy-tale moment when you realize that your whole life before motherhood was meaningless. It's normal for new mothers to feel a sense of loss: loss of their old, premotherhood identity, loss of their former career if they don't plan to return to work, and loss of the freedom and independence they once knew.

Frustration and Boredom

You may find yourself growing frustrated by not being able to plan your own schedule, or bored with the day-to-day routine of caring for a little person's needs. This is normal and doesn't mean you aren't a good mother, or that you don't love your baby. It also doesn't mean that you won't eventually get used to your new role. With time, you will start to feel bits and pieces of your old life creeping back in, and you'll become adept at balancing your baby with the other things you want to accomplish. Just take the time to enjoy and get to know your baby: the rest will wait, but he'll only be this small once.

Essential

Many moms are using blogs—short for "Web log"—to write about the ins and outs of motherhood. Check out *www.dot-moms.com* to read what other moms have to say about raising kids—both the joys and the hard parts. You may be inspired to start a blog of your own.

It's Okay to Be "Just a Mom"

Some women, on the other hand, adjust quite easily to motherhood. You may find that you're not eager to return to work, or if you're planning on staying home with the baby, that you don't miss your prebaby life at all. This is also normal, and doesn't mean that the "old you" is gone. Caring for a baby can be fun, exciting, and fulfilling, and it's totally understandable if you find yourself immersed in the little world your baby and you create together.

A Mixed Bag

And sometimes, you'll find yourself wavering between two worlds: intense love for your baby and satisfaction in mothering tasks like diapering and feeding, mixed with intermittent boredom, anxiety, or even anger. This is also normal. New motherhood is an incredibly intense, emotion-filled time, and there's no way to predict what you will feel from one moment to the next.

Bonding with Your Baby

Many people describe bonding as a magical moment that happens at the moment of your baby's birth, when you're overcome by love for this little person. While that's certainly the way it happens for a lot of women, not all mothers feel that immediate sense of connection—sometimes, that love bond takes a while to grow. And even if you did feel an immediate rush of joy and elation when you saw your baby, you may have doubts during your first weeks of motherhood— am I doing this right? Am I bonding strongly enough with my baby? Am I giving him *too much* attention?

L. Essential

Even if you'd already planned on going back to work or staying home before your baby was born, you may find that the decision is more complicated now that he's actually here. It's okay to change your mind. Do what you think is best for you, your baby, and your family now.

How Babies Bond

Babies and mothers bond with all their senses. Your baby is learning to love your smell, the sound of your voice, the feel of your skin, the sight of your face, and the taste of your milk. You may find yourself wanting to smell, touch, look at, hear, and maybe even taste him, too! It's normal—enjoy it!

Can You Love Your Baby Too Much?

It's natural to want to hold your baby all the time, to not want to be separated from him, and to not want to hear him cry. Babies are programmed to get adult attention from their cries, and mothers are hard-wired to respond to their babies' needs. Through touch and attention to his needs, your baby will learn to trust you, and you'll forge an even stronger bond with him.

Fact

A recent study conducted by the University of London showed that when parents don't respond to their young babies' cries, the babies cry 50 percent more—and continue to cry more at twelve weeks of age.

Feeling a Sense of Accomplishment

One of the hardest things about adjusting to motherhood can be taking control of your time. What used to be a quick and easy chore, like making the bed or folding laundry, can now seem to take hours between feedings, diaper changes, and walking a crying baby around the room. You may feel like everything around you is falling into disarray, while all the plans you made for how you'd spend your postpartum "vacation" get buried under a stack of unwashed dishes.

Let Some Things Go

As mentioned previously, it's not always easy to put the perfectionist side of yourself on hold, but you absolutely must give yourself a break during this time. To meet your baby's needs and still have your hands free to get a few things done, get a good sling that holds your baby close to your body. Of course, be careful while wearing your baby around hot stoves or other potential dangers.

Make Lists of Manageable Tasks

Breaking tasks down into manageable chunks can help you feel like you're getting something accomplished. Instead of thinking "Today I'll clean the kitchen," think "I'd like to wipe the countertops, wipe down the fridge and stove, and sweep the floor." Write down each step on a piece of paper. That way, if your baby gives you a minute, you can attack one of these tasks and then cross it off the list—proof that you are, in fact, getting things done.

Your Mothering Style

Are you a free-thinking earth mother or a rigid scheduler? Magazine articles, TV shows, and sometimes other parents often seem eager to slap labels on mothers, maybe as a way of pitting mom against mom. But by labeling yourself this or that kind of mom, you take the chance of setting your expectations so high you can't meet them. Also, you may find that your baby's actual personality or your actual life don't mesh very well with the image of yourself you'd been holding in your head. And if you hold too judgmentally to certain ideas and ideals, you risk missing out on friendships you might have had with other moms who don't measure up to the unreachable standard you've created.

⌊ Essential

For many mothers, wearing their babies goes beyond convenience and becomes a lifestyle. Slings and baby carriers can make parenting high-needs babies more manageable and promote a strong attachment between you and your little one. For more information about carrying and "wearing" babies in a sling, check out ✎www .thebabywearer.com.

Be Flexible

Every mother holds certain issues and traits near and dear to her heart. But your baby is a unique individual who might not conform to your ideas about what babies should and shouldn't do. This can be frustrating to mothers who, for example, thought they would have their babies on a strict feeding schedule, only to find that the baby is miserable on a schedule and cries all the time. Or, the mother who dreams of co-sleeping with her baby, only to find that he sleeps a lot better alone. No matter what kind of parent you think you'll be, chances are good that your baby will find at least one way to challenge your expectations. Don't throw your ideas about parenting out the window, but do be flexible and open minded. Follow your instincts, and reserve the right to change your mind.

Alert

Most moms have to deal with somebody criticizing their parenting style sooner or later, and the criticism can really undermine your confidence. Just remember, you are your baby's mother, and you know best. It may help to only discuss child-rearing topics with supportive friends and family. Eventually you'll be able to take dissent in stride.

Nobody's Perfect

It's important to remember that parenthood is a whole, not the sum of its parts. You can and will make mistakes, and your baby will still thrive—no mother is perfect. Sometimes, you will have to weigh your baby's needs against the needs of the whole family and come up with a compromise. As your baby grows, you will become more confident and sure about following your gut. In the meantime, remember: you and your baby are in this together, and you'll learn from each other as you go.

Caring for Yourself

You've been a lot of things in your life: daughter, student, wife, and employee. But probably none have threatened to upset all the rest like your role of mother. Being a new mom can be so all-encompassing that you feel like you've lost the rest of yourself in the balance. The "old you" is still there, and will be with you long after your baby grows up.

Though motherhood requires sacrifice, it's important not to cross the line into martyrdom. You need to take care of yourself as well as your baby, with nutritious food, adequate rest, and some time to yourself to talk with friends, meditate, write, read, or whatever activities you enjoy that leave you feeling refreshed and balanced. Don't feel guilty about leaving the baby with your partner and taking an hour or two for yourself once in a while. Your baby needs a happy, healthy mother, and it will be good for your partner and your baby to get to know each other without your being there to bail them out. If he has to, your partner will get the hang of comforting and calming a cranky baby, and you can rest easier knowing that if you have an errand to run in the future, your baby will be in competent and confident hands.

Every mom needs a break now and then, but the hassle and worry that can be involved with leaving a nursing baby at home sometimes makes it more trouble than it's worth to go out. If that's the case, maybe your partner can help you arrange an evening in. You can have friends over for a movie, a drink, or a game of cards, while he and the baby retreat to another area of the house. You'll be able to relax and have fun with your friends, but still be accessible in case the baby gets hungry. And you'll probably be feeling refreshed enough to return the favor, so it's a win-win.

Your Social Network

Motherhood can be isolating, and new moms are often shocked by how demanding their new role is. "I didn't know it would be like this" is a common cry of a bewildered new mother, trying to keep afloat as she navigates the rocky new waters she's found herself in. A social support system is absolutely vital to your emotional and even physical health as a new mom. Research has shown that mothers given adequate social support during childbirth have better outcomes and shorter labors and that they interact with their babies more. Other research has linked health and life expectancy to the quality of social connections. It's reasonable to deduce, then, that moms who have a good support community will be healthier emotionally and physically as new mothers, and that they'll be better and more engaged mothers as well.

⌐ Essential

Looking for other moms in your area? Try logging on to ✑*www* *.mamasource.com*, a site that connects moms living in the same area for friendship, advice, and referrals to health-care providers, babysitters, and other services families need.

Unless you have a large circle of friends who are having kids around the same time as you, you may find yourself spending your days alone, wondering what the outside world is doing and trying to figure out how to be a part of it. Your single friends are probably working during the day and going out at night, and may be unsure of how to include you in their lives now that you've got a baby.

Your Old Friends

If the invitations have stopped rolling in from your friends who don't have kids, it may just be that they don't think you'd be interested in having lunch or going out for a drink now that you've got a baby—even if that's the furthest thing from the truth. If your best pals love babies, you may have no trouble convincing them that you're just as much fun—maybe even more fun—with your new sidekick around. Eventually, those friends who want children will probably be glad they've been able to watch and learn from you as a parent.

Friends without kids can be great. Everything is new and novel to them, so chances are good that they'll find your baby just as fascinating as you do. Childless friends often love to "borrow" babies for fun and practice. They can keep you connected to that side of yourself that's still carefree and independent.

But if you have friends who aren't sure how they feel about kids, they may be uncertain about including you in social events. If they invite the baby too, will they have to listen to crying? If you come without the baby, will you bore everyone with tales of teething and poop?

Let your old friends know that you're still the same person, even if you are spending a lot of your time with someone lacking scintillating conversation skills. Invite friends over for a drink after you know the baby will be asleep for the night. Keep in mind that, though some friends may be eager for every developmental detail, others may not want to rehash drooling and diapering for hours.

When Old Friendships Die

Be prepared, though, that some of your old friendships just may not survive your journey into motherhood. If you're missing your old life, keeping connections with your prebaby friends can be helpful, unless your get-togethers end with you feeling like your new life isn't as interesting or meaningful as theirs. If you feel like a friendship is imploding, try not to take it personally: an old friend may not understand or value your new priorities or may be jealous of you, or you may simply be growing apart.

Finding Supportive Friends

It's important that your mothering groups are supportive and understanding of your parenting style and that you feel your mothering skills are valued within the group. You needn't agree 100 percent with the other mothers about every parenting issue, but knowing that they respect and support you as a mother is vital. But don't fall into the trap of only seeking out people who parent exactly the way you do, or who are the same age or at roughly the same place on the parenting journey as you are. More experienced mothers can act as mentors, and can offer proof that you, too, will come through this confusing period just fine, while befriending greener moms will put you in the role of mentor, which allows you to give back and can give your self-esteem a boost. And you can learn from and be gently challenged by the perspectives of mothers who (respectfully) parent differently than you do.

Tools that Will Make Your Life Easier

Beyond the basics, babies really don't need a lot of gear to thrive. This is great news, especially since your finances might now be stretched more than ever before. But not all baby products are meant exclusively for the baby—some tools can make a mother's life a lot easier. More expensive products are a bit of an investment, but getting what you need and paying for high quality is usually worth it in the long run.

A Good Sling or Baby Carrier

Don't buy a cheap version of a sling or baby carrier from the discount or department store—they often don't provide your back or neck with enough support and are difficult to get in and out of. The Baby Bjorn front carrier, Maya Wrap baby sling, and the Moby Wrap sling are all popular tried-and-true carrier and sling brands you can purchase in specialty shops, through catalogs, or online. There are plenty of styles out there, so look around online for one that looks good to you. Keep in mind that when it comes to slings, styles with padding are sometimes more comfortable, but are harder to stuff in a bag or wear under a coat; ring styles are more adjustable but often have extra fabric; and pouch styles are easy-on, easy-off, but don't allow you to tighten or loosen the sling for a better fit. If you don't want to pay full price, check consignment stores and eBay. You may want a couple of kinds of slings for different occasions.

A Slow Cooker

Fill a slow cooker with food in the morning, turn it on, leave it all day, and eat at night. Slow cookers can make a variety of meals from soups and chili to dips to slow-cooked meats, and they make meal planning manageable for even the most stressed-out mom. There are lots of great cookbooks out there that have recipes tailored specifically to the slow cooker. You can also refrigerate or freeze leftovers for quick and easy meals to eat days later.

A Central Calendar

Now that you've got not only you and your husband's schedules to keep track of but also doctor's visits, shot records, mother's group meetings, the babysitter's phone number, and a million other baby-related nuggets of information, you're going to need a place to write all this information down. A calendar that both you and your partner check daily can help the two of you stay up-to-date when it comes to appointments and the like. You can use an interactive online calendar that both of you can access from your own computers, like the one at *www.google.com/calendar*, or just hang a regular paper calendar in a central area, like the kitchen. A calendar with an attached dry-erase board will give you a place to scribble notes to each other, whether it's "I love you" or "Need more milk."

A Good Stroller

Any stroller will get you and your baby around town, but a really good stroller can make walks to the park much more enjoyable. Cup holders, a sunshade and rain bonnet, a roomy basket, a handle that reaches far enough up so you don't have to bend over to reach it, wheels that can handle a variety of terrains and absorb shock, and a feature that allows the stroller to fold down easily so you can throw it in the back of the car are all features that can mean the difference between getting where you have to go and strolling in comfort and style.

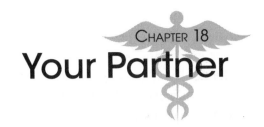

CHAPTER 18

Your Partner

HAVING A BABY IS a wonderful thing, but you might not have been prepared for the way it would change your relationships. It's common for men and women to go through disagreements and differences as they learn to juggle home, finances, work, and their partner with the huge responsibility of raising a child. Some differences of opinion are to be expected, but if you communicate with understanding and work to stay connected, you can come through parenthood with your partnership even stronger than it was before.

Your Partner's Feelings

Men and women often deal with the stresses of parenting differently. While you may be worrying about feeding and caring for your baby properly, chances are good that your partner is dealing with another list of fears. With a lot of your attention being focused on the baby, for example, he may be feeling left out or ignored. He may also be worrying about practical matters like money and balancing work with family time.

Money

There's a good chance your spouse is worried about finances: how much parenthood will cost, and if you'll be able to get by financially. This can be compounded if you don't plan to return to work right away or will be staying at home for the foreseeable future. Money is one of the largest stressors in a marriage, so it's important to make sure you're on the same page. Try to ease his fears by sitting down and planning out your finances on paper. Have a plan; if not working will put you in debt or if you'll have to use some of your savings, show how the two of you can make up for it in other ways. Also, encourage your husband to be realistic about how much babies cost—figures like $100,000 per child get thrown around a lot, but there are lifestyle choices you can make like breastfeeding, thrift-store shopping, and cloth diapering that can save money and lower that estimate considerably.

Sometimes at-home mothers feel guilty, like they're spending their partner's money. They may have a hard time asking for money for things they want or even things the family needs. Keep in mind that your partner's earnings aren't his money—the money is there to support your whole family. You are doing an important job by caring for your baby—that's your contribution to the family. Regardless of whose name is on the paycheck, you and your partner have an equal say in what happens to your family's income, and should be making financial decisions together.

Essential

If you have to work, but aren't crazy about the idea—or expense—of day care, consider working a shift opposite that of your partner. If you're saving the cost of child care, one of you may be able to work fewer hours without reducing your family's disposable income.

If you and your partner are having financial disagreements, it might be helpful to sit down and make a list of financial and life goals. Maybe your misunderstandings are being caused by differing ideas about what role money should play in your family's life. Understanding each other's values will help you compromise.

Being Left Out

Many new dads worry that once the baby comes, you won't have any time left for him. It's true that in the early days postpartum, your relationship with your baby takes center stage, and that can be worrisome to your partner if he thinks he'll be the third wheel from here on out. Find ways to involve him with your baby's care from day one. Feeding isn't everything—if you're nursing, he can still rock the baby to sleep, take care of diaper changes, and give the baby his bath. And if you get your baby used to Daddy putting him to sleep early on, that job won't always have to fall to you in the future. In the early weeks, you may have a hard time doing much besides feeding your baby, but you can still find time to chat with your husband about his day or watch a favorite TV program together. And as your baby gets older and caring for him is a little less intense, be sure to add back some of the things you and your partner did together before the baby was born. You can still go to dinner or take a long walk together, even if you do have a small sidekick with you.

Loss of Freedom

Weekend trips with the guys, grabbing a beer on the way home from work . . . yes, for a new dad, these are probably off the agenda—at least for a while. But your partner may worry that his days of after-hours fun are over now that you've got a baby. While it's true that being a dad means making sacrifices, parenthood doesn't have to mean an end to independent fun forever—for either one of you.

 Alert

Sometimes, too much togetherness can strain your relationship. Instead of insisting you and your husband do everything together, you may find it refreshing for both of you to have a friend over on a Friday night and send your partner out with his friends instead. Next time, it'll be your turn to go out while he stays in.

No More Sex?

Your partner is probably worried about what the baby is going to mean for your sex life. And the harsh truth is that your sex life will be different from what it was like before you had a baby.

But you can help put your partner's mind at ease by letting him know that, even though you may be feeling less-than-sexy for the next few months, you don't anticipate a life of celibacy. See Chapter 16 for tips on keeping your sex life afloat while you've got a new baby.

Being a Good Dad

Unless your partner was raised the oldest of a slew of siblings, he may not have had an opportunity to learn about caring for babies. While teenage girls are often indoctrinated in baby care through babysitting and instruction from older women, adults don't always think to pass those skills on to boys.

Essential

Babysitting or attending a parenting class together before your baby is born is a good way for your partner to learn some basic baby-care skills like diapering and bathing. Some childbirth education classes also offer a baby-care component.

If your partner is intimidated by your baby, the best way to help him feel more comfortable is by letting him care for the baby. Don't interfere or "help" unless he asks for it—in fact, to avoid giving him performance anxiety, it might be best to hand the baby over and go take a nap or a bubble bath. With time and opportunity, your partner will become confident in his skills and more willing to take over for you for longer periods of time.

Balancing a Job and a Family

If your partner's job keeps him at the office for long hours or if he travels a lot, he may be worried that he won't be able to be there to watch his baby grow. Nowadays, it's becoming more and more common for dads to leave high-pressure jobs with long hours to pursue something more family friendly.

 Fact

Many companies are required to offer twelve weeks of unpaid paternity leave under the Family and Medical Leave Act. If you can afford it, extended paternity leave can give you and your partner a gentle transition into parenthood and allow you both plenty of time to get to know your baby.

It can be hard to break free of those pesky traditional gender roles, but keep your husband's feelings and needs in mind. If he wants to leave a high-paying job for something a little less lucrative and you're worried how that might affect your lifestyle, ask yourself this question: how would you want your partner to react if you wanted to take a less-stressful job that would allow you to spend more time with your baby?

Parenting Disagreements

From time to time you and your partner are bound to have disagreements about parenting, whether it's a feeding, disciplining, or even diapering issue. Moms sometimes feel entitled to make all the decisions—after all, she's the one who went through pregnancy and birth!—and may also feel more emotionally invested in whether a baby is fed, changed, or put to bed in a certain way. Dads may not be sure where they fit in when it comes to decision-making and may become resentful if it feels like his opinions don't matter.

You're never going to agree on everything, but it's important that you communicate, compromise, and when possible, be consistent in your approach. As your baby grows, he'll quickly learn whether

Mom and Dad are on the same team, or whether he can play them against one another to get what he wants. It's crucial that you work out how to come to parenting decisions together early on so that you can present a unified front.

L. Essential

When you and your partner discuss parenting disagreements, keep his personality in mind. Does he respond best to anecdotal evidence or scientific research? Just because he doesn't agree at first doesn't mean he won't be receptive to an idea if you present it in a way that speaks to him.

Keeping Communication Strong

No matter how tired or frustrated you are, the biggest keys to coming through this period with your relationship strongly intact are communication and compassion. Don't stop talking to each other—that's how little things add up and turn into big trouble.

First of all, if you don't clear the air regularly, that annoying little thing he did last week (like forgetting to clean the diaper pail) can fester under the surface until it becomes a Very Big Deal in your mind. Also try approaching disagreements without attacking or being passive-aggressive. Saying "You never help around the house!" is more likely to cause a defensive reaction or a fight than the less accusatory "I feel frustrated when I've been up all night with the baby and see that the dinner dishes are still on the table." Keep your complaints on point—don't bring up the time he blew off dinner with you so he could stay late at the office a year ago. It may feel relevant, but it won't help the current discussion about what needs to be fixed in your house right now. And more than one mother has complained that loud sighs, slamming doors, and stomping around the house doesn't do much to get her partner's attention, either. The key is directness without too much drama.

Keep in mind that both of you are probably on edge: tired, stressed, and anxious. Try to be forgiving of one another's snappy comebacks and sarcasm. If you approach each conversation assuming that the other person has good intentions, it's easier to avoid common communication traps and to keep resentment from taking hold.

Making Time for Each Other

You've probably been advised to go on regular dates with your husband to keep your relationship strong—and keep the romance alive. But working around a baby's feeding schedule, paying for the cost of a sitter and an evening out, and the uncertainty over leaving the baby with someone new can take all the fun out of what is supposed to be a relaxing time with your spouse.

If you can't or don't want to leave your baby just yet, you can still go on regular "dates" with your partner—it just takes some creativity. Some ways to stay connected:

- **Enjoy a romantic dinner in the late evening, after the baby's gone to bed.** While one of you sets the mood with candles, music, and maybe a roaring fire, the other can call your favorite restaurant to have a meal prepared for pickup.
- **Rent past seasons of a TV show you both love, and watch one episode together each night.** That way, you can watch the show when the baby's not likely to interrupt, and use the pause button as needed.
- **Any shared activity can help keep your bond strong.** If you enjoy being active, try biking, hiking, or hiking with the baby in a backpack, trailer, or stroller once you've gotten the go-ahead from your doctor or midwife. Some couples enjoy training for 5K runs or other competitions together. If you're into more sedentary activities, play cards or a board game together. If you enjoy art or history, put the baby in a sling and head out to a gallery or museum.

The point is to make time for each other every day to talk and stay connected. You don't have to hire a sitter and spend an evening in an expensive restaurant to get the benefits of a date night, though sometimes that can be nice too. The more connected you feel, the easier it will be to communicate with patience and understanding.

Who's Doing the Housework?

One common fight new moms and dads have is how to divide the household chores. Though most women are now employed outside the home, men and women often find themselves falling into traditional gender roles in their off-hours, meaning the women do the vast majority of the housework.

A Baby Changes Things

The woman doing the bulk of household work might be manageable or even go mostly unnoticed early in a marriage, but add a baby and suddenly the inequality of the situation becomes much more obvious. Faced with the new role of caring for a baby 24 hours, 7 days a week—often while sleep deprived—a woman may find herself unable and unwilling to also do all the cooking, cleaning, and managing of the household tasks. During the first six weeks, you should be resting and getting to know your baby, and household tasks will naturally fall by the wayside. After the six-week mark, you may be readying yourself to go back to work. Even if you'll be at home with the baby, it will be impossible to keep up with everything the way you did before and take good care of your baby and yourself. If your partner didn't help keep the house running before you had the baby, things will have to change now.

Tell Him What You Need

But don't assume that his seeming lack of enthusiasm over housework stems from laziness or that he doesn't care about your feelings and needs. Your partner may want to help out, but he may not be sure exactly how to do it. He may also not see messes with the same critical eye as you do, so it may not be obvious to him that a sinkful of dishes means that somebody should wash them. Keep in mind that you may have to be very specific—just because he did the dishes yesterday, don't assume he'll think to do them again today. A gentle nonaccusatory reminder will help you get what you want (the dishes done today, too) without making him defensive.

Essential

While traditionally women do more of the household chores, in some marriages it's the other way around. If your husband has been the person handling most of the cleaning, keep in mind that he's got other priorities now, too. You'll need to relax your standards and, when you're feeling up to it, chip in with tasks that he can't do on his own.

Lower Standards

You may both have to relax your expectations when it comes to housework. If you're doing all you can and your spouse doesn't think the house is clean enough, he should be willing to pick up the slack to get things up to his standards. On the other hand, while you should definitely expect your partner to pitch in with cleaning, when he gets home from work he'd probably rather play with the baby. Instead of struggling with trying to keep the house clean all day while taking care of your baby at the same time, maybe you can hand off the baby when your husband gets home and do a quick tidy-up. After you're done, you can take the baby back and he can take care of his household tasks. When you work together it shouldn't take long to whip the house into something that's at least livable, if not perfect.

Make a Task List

Tracking who does what for a week can be a useful way to figure out if the balance is off in your household. Don't think of it as keeping score; use it instead as a way of determining how often certain chores need to be done, when, and who might be the logical person to handle them. For example, it might be easier for you to do a load of dishes with the baby in a sling than it is to carry a full laundry basket up and down the stairs. If you know that you don't have to worry about the laundry, you may feel less overwhelmed when faced with the dishes. Or, if there are certain tasks you really hate, maybe your spouse can take over those so you don't have to worry about them. Keep in mind that a partnership is rarely truly 50-50. The balance doesn't always have to be perfect, as long as both partners are dedicated to helping each other, and both are satisfied with the arrangement.

L, Essential

Have you ever heard the expression "work smarter, not harder"? If you find you're devoting a lot of time to dusting knick-knacks and trying to find baby photos under piles of clutter, you may need to work together to find ways to eliminate extra work, by temporarily boxing up and storing things you can't take care of right now or investing in convenient cleaning supplies and devices.

And don't forget about those unseen aspects of baby care and household management. In many households, keeping track of doctor and dentist visits often fall to Mom by default, while dads handle all the finances. In reality, it's better if both of you participate in both of these areas, at least to some degree: you need to understand what's happening with the family's money and help make choices about it, and if you're both involved in your baby's medical care, you'll be able to make health-related decisions together. That can take the pressure off of both of you.

Plan, Plan, Plan

Once you have a rough idea of who's going to do what, figure out when it's going to happen. Be specific: if you know your husband's planning to do the dishes at 9:00 after he's finished watching TV, you won't spend the evening feeling antsy wondering if you're going to wake up to a messy kitchen the next day. And if you've mapped out your meals ahead of time, you'll know which days you have kitchen duties, which days your husband will be cooking, and better yet, when you can order pizza.

Be Flexible

It's not always easy to foresee every obstacle ahead of time. Maybe your husband thought he'd be able to get up early and make breakfast every morning, but he's paying for losing sleep by having trouble focusing at work. Or maybe you expected that you'd be able to vacuum the living room every day, but as it turns out, the baby is terrified of the vacuum. Make a date to sit down and review your plan every so often and see how it's going. If it's not working for either of you, it's time to come up with something new.

Be Open to Nontraditional Roles

Maybe you're at home, but would really rather be working, while your husband pines away for home from his office all day. Outdated cultural norms that dictate that men should be the primary breadwinners while women should keep the home fires burning can get in the way of your real desires and strengths as a partnership. If you're better at managing the money, there's no reason why you shouldn't be in charge of the checkbook. If you hate cooking and your husband is a passionate cook, there's no reason why he can't do most of the food preparation. And a growing number of dads are either leaving their jobs or reducing their hours to be the primary at-home parent. Taking on a role you aren't suited for just because it's what you think you should do won't make anyone happy. When you and your partner talk about possibilities for dividing up work and duties, don't limit yourself to "men's work" and "women's work."

Postpartum Depression for Dads?

Recent research from the University of Oxford indicates that men can also suffer from a form of postpartum depression, and the symptoms—lack of energy, sleeplessness, anxiety and worry, fatigue, and weight gain, to name a few—can look a lot like the symptoms of a woman's postpartum depression. If your partner seems withdrawn, isn't participating in caring for the baby, is angry or irritable, or can't seem to get off of the couch, it's possible he's depressed. Depressed fathers can lead to behavioral problems in young children, and new mothers need the support of an engaged partner, so if you worry that your spouse might be depressed, it's a good idea to seek help. Both of you might benefit from therapy. If your spouse won't go to counseling, you can go by yourself to learn how to cope.

CHAPTER 19

Special Circumstances

EVERY MOTHER'S POSTPARTUM EXPERIENCE is different, but single moms, those whose babies are sick or premature, those who gave their babies up for adoption, or those whose babies have died face special obstacles and have different needs when it comes to emotional and physical recovery. This chapter offers tips, tools, and resources that will help you take good care of yourself if your circumstances aren't quite typical.

Single Moms

If you had a baby alone by choice or by chance, you're probably already acutely aware that advice like "Ask your partner to do more housework" won't help you—there's only one of you to do all the work of raising a baby, paying the bills, and keeping the house from falling down. But even without a partner to help, single mothers can not only survive, but thrive.

Preparation

If you have time to prepare before your baby is born, there's a lot you can do to make your postpartum period easier. For example, if you want to apply for any programs like Medicaid, child care assistance, or WIC (Women, Infants, and Children, which provides food to pregnant and nursing mothers and babies), get as much of the paperwork and documentation together before your baby is born so there will be less to do postpartum.

Alert

If possible, consult with a lawyer before your baby is born to get a clear understanding of your rights and responsibilities. If you can't afford a lawyer's fees, a local law school may offer free or low-cost legal advice. Or see if your area has a Legal Aid clinic.

If the baby's father will be involved, you'll want to discuss some specifics ahead of time—when will he be visiting the baby? What kind of visitation and custody arrangements will he seek? What about child support? All these considerations can be very stressful, and you don't want to be dealing with any surprises or battles right after your baby is born.

If You Weren't Ready for This

Some mothers become unexpectedly single very close to their due dates or right after the baby's born. In those situations, you may need to lean heavily on close friends and family—perhaps even spending some time living with your parents or another loved one while you're recovering. Try not to worry about anything besides you and your baby at this time. Let others care for you. Becoming suddenly single is stressful enough; trying to care for a baby alone adds a whole new level of strain.

Your Baby's Father

Depending on your relationship, your baby's father might be a source of support and encouragement during this time, or your interactions with him may cause you stress, anger, pain, and fear. All of those emotions can be taxing and are not something you need to be dealing with during your postpartum weeks. If you find that contact with your baby's father is just too stressful for you but you still want to give him access to the baby, try finding a third party to act as the intermediary, somebody who can bring the baby to him and then bring the baby back to you. You could even do this in your own home if you have a place where he can get comfortable while visiting the baby while you retreat to your bedroom or take a bath.

 ## Fact

In most states, mothers are typically granted physical custody of their newborn babies until other arrangements are worked out in court, which takes time. You probably won't have to worry about custody battles right off the bat. That means you have a certain amount of control over the situation.

If you do have any trouble with your baby's father during the postpartum period, document everything. The two of you may not see eye-to-eye on every issue, but if your interactions with him start to affect your sleep or make you overly anxious and stressed out, it's probably best to put off difficult discussions until the baby is a little older. All the details don't have to be nailed down right away. If your baby's father is putting a lot of pressure on you, it may be best to turn interactions over to an attorney to keep you from experiencing additional stress.

Help from Friends or Relatives

Don't underestimate how tired and sore you might be after your baby is born. It's a good idea to arrange for a close friend or relative, like your sister or mother, to stay with you for as long as possible after your baby is born. Even if you're feeling well after giving birth, you'll want to stay in bed and rest as much as possible and shouldn't be cooking, cleaning, or attending to older children. And having an extra set of arms to hold the baby while you shower or to bring you a glass of water while you're nursing can be very helpful. If you have a c-section, you'll absolutely need hands-on help as you're recovering from surgery. You can also stay with a parent or friend for a while if they can accommodate both you and your baby comfortably. Whoever you ask, make sure it's someone who you have a good and uncomplicated relationship with, and somebody who will support you as a parent. You don't want to put yourself in the position of defending your mothering choices or feeling tense and anxious about someone who's supposed to be helping take care of you.

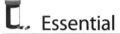 Essential

> If you know you're going to be a single mom, consider attending—or starting—a support group for single parents before your baby's born. You may find that you need a strong support community the most in the early weeks, when it can be difficult to reach out.

Professional Help

Some single moms find that they don't mind the solitude at all—on the contrary, they're glad to be able to focus completely on their baby without having to worry about interacting with anyone else. Others don't have any family or friends they'd feel comfortable bringing into their home for a long period of time, or don't have anyone willing or available to help out. If you don't want or can't get any live-in help, keep in mind that it is very difficult to take care of your own needs when you don't have anyone else to lean on. If you can, consider hiring help like a postpartum doula or a cleaning service to pick up some of the slack, and reach out to your social network for friendship and support.

A Single Mom's Emotional Life

Single moms are at a higher risk of developing postpartum depression, and for good reason: parenting is hard work, and it's doubly hard when you don't have a partner to help with the emotional and physical work. Still, there are ways you can cope with the emotional difficulties of single motherhood.

Rethink Your Idea of "Family"

If your family doesn't look like the wife, husband, and baby down the street, it's easy to feel lonely and inadequate. But by reworking your mental picture of what a "family" is, you can find new ways to reach out to the people already in your life. For instance, if you're feeling bad about not having a partner to share your baby's development with, you could ask a close friend to act as a milestone buddy, so that when your baby has a special achievement, you'll have someone you can call who can't wait to gush over the good news.

 Question

> **Can I really raise a happy, healthy child as a single parent?**
> The news seems full of unsettling statistics about the kids of single parents. But you are not a statistic. With support, planning, and flexibility, you can provide your baby with a stable, happy, loving childhood.

Focus on the Moment

Try focusing on what you do have instead of what you don't have. Thinking forward to a time when things might be easier can be helpful, but not if it makes you anxious or keeps you from appreciating the way your baby looks, feels, and smells right now. Try to be fully present and enjoy your baby. If the rest of the house is falling down around you, that can be fixed later. Don't think too much about what's down the road or what mistakes, challenges, or obstacles you might face tomorrow, next week, or next month. Take it one day, hour, or minute at a time—whatever helps you cope.

Know Things Will Improve

Don't fixate on the future, but do remember that things will continue to get better. Your body will begin to get back to normal, and your baby will sleep longer stretches at a time, eventually through the night. You'll start to feel up to getting out and doing some of the things you used to love.

Find Your Tribe

Everything feels harder when you're doing it alone. When you're parenting your baby alongside a friend or group of supportive moms, you may find that the more tedious tasks that can threaten to overwhelm you when you're by yourself, like constant diapering and feeding, seem much more manageable. Chatting and sharing the workload with a group of mothers can feel refreshing and rejuvenating. Also, a group of like-minded moms gives you a place to turn with questions or concerns about parenting.

Don't feel like you need to limit your mom's group activity to sitting around a circle chatting. There are plenty of ways you can help one another and benefit from your mom friends. Here are some ideas:

- Get together with another mom on the weekend and cook and freeze meals for the upcoming week.
- Do your grocery shopping with a friend. That way, if one of you has to temporarily remove a screaming baby, the other can watch her grocery cart. You can also help each other load and unload groceries.
- Cleaning is much more manageable—and enjoyable—with a friend. Take turns getting together to clean one person's house thoroughly, then swap houses. You can focus on one room at a time—say, organize each others' hall closets one week, then deep-clean the bathrooms another.
- Dinner for one person and a baby can be lonely. Why not regularly get together for dinner with another single mom and her kids?

Where the Moms Are

Check churches, community centers, and organizations like La Leche League, Mommy and Me, and MOPS (Mothers of Preschoolers) for parenting support groups. If you don't find what you're looking for, start your own group. Ask your doctor or midwife if he or she can help connect you with local single moms or moms-to-be. Mom-baby yoga and fitness classes can also be a great way to meet other mothers. You can also ask about posting fliers at the library, in your doctor's office, or on college campuses.

Many local support groups also communicate via e-mail lists. Two popular e-mail list services are Yahoo! Groups at *http://groups.yahoo.com* and Google groups at *http://groups.google.com*. Search these e-mail list services for mothering groups in your area, or start your own. Moms looking for support groups online may find you and join the list.

Multiples

Two or more babies at once can mean twice the joy, but it can also mean twice the fatigue and work. It also means that your body produced a higher level of hormones during pregnancy, which can mean a greater risk of postpartum depression and blues when the hormones fluctuate after your baby is born.

Breastfeeding Multiples

Many women breastfeed multiple babies successfully—often nursing two at the same time. It requires dedication, but if you're committed to making it work, you can. It's a good idea to get help, preferably from the first day, from a lactation consultant, La Leche League volunteer, or friend who's experienced with nursing twins.

Surviving the Daily Grind

Moms with newborn twins are often exhausted and may feel like they do nothing but hold and feed their babies all day. No doubt about it, taking care of more than one baby takes plenty of patience and energy, but there are some things you can do to make parenting multiples easier on yourself:

- Adjust your expectations. It's impossible to care for two (or more) newborns and also keep a clean house, make home-cooked meals, and get out all those thank-you cards. Simplify your life and realize that, for now, some things simply aren't going to get done unless they're absolutely essential.
- Learn the tricks of the trade. Get together with other moms of multiples (or find them online) to learn how they get things done. Visit *http://multiples.about.com* for ideas and resources.
- When you've got two babies, chances are good at least one of them will be in arms most of the time. Learning to wear two babies in slings at the same time can be a lifesaver. You can also wear one baby while the other spends some time in a bouncy seat, and switch back and forth every so often. Double strollers are another good investment.
- Keep everything nearby and accessible. Keep baskets with everything you might need for the babies' care (and your care, too) in different areas of the house so that, once you're in one room, you don't have to run around the house to grab diapers, wipes, the phone, a bottle of water, etc.
- Focus on your life as it is right now. One day, you'll be able to keep a clean house again, but for today, it may be enough just to make sure everybody's fed (that includes you).
- Don't feel guilty about eating convenience foods. Something has to give, and home-cooked meals are probably off the agenda for several months—at least. Fruit, nuts, bagged salads, turkey sandwiches on whole-wheat bread, and whole-grain cold cereal may not be gourmet meals, but they're all relatively healthy foods that take little or no time to prepare.
- Learn some deep breathing, visualization, or meditation exercises you can use while stressed. Stress is a contributor

to postpartum depression, and you'll have multiple stressors, not to mention multiple reasons for sleep deprivation.

 Alert

With multiples, it can be more difficult to get enough sleep, drink enough water, and eat well enough, which can make it more difficult to produce enough milk. If you don't think you're making enough milk, make sure your breasts are getting stimulated often and that you're eating well, drinking, and resting.

Finally, continually remind yourself that there is no such thing as a "perfect" mother or a "right" way to raise multiples. Observe your children and let their health and happiness—and your own—be your guide.

If You Had a Traumatic Birth

Traumatic birth experiences can not only make your physical recovery more difficult, but can also leave you feeling confused, sad, angry, and anxious. You are probably going to need the help of both professionals and loved ones to help you work through any remaining negative feelings you may be experiencing.

Physical Concerns

Traumatic births can lead to a variety of physical outcomes, from a damaged pelvic floor due to use of forceps to anemia from blood loss or the after-effects of general anesthesia. If you experienced birth injuries, you may have to take extra-good care of yourself and allow others to do everything for you as you recover. Even the stress involved in a frightening birth experience can have an effect on your physical recovery.

Emotional Responses

Traumatic birth experiences sometimes lead to a delay in bonding. You may be so physically exhausted by your baby's birth that you need some time to collect yourself, or you may have been too sick or woozy to pay much attention to your baby after he was born. This can lead to feelings of guilt and regret later, and you might wonder if you would have a stronger relationship with your baby if your birth had gone differently.

Birth trauma can also lead to mourning for the birth you might have had. If your baby is healthy, people around you may not understand why you're grieving over your birth experience. But birth can be enormously important. It is your introduction to motherhood, and if your birth was traumatic, you may feel uncertain about your role as a mother, victimized by your caregivers, or even resentful of your baby.

 Alert

Sometimes, a very difficult or frightening birth can lead to severe postpartum depression or even postpartum posttraumatic stress disorder (PTSD). For more information on postpartum depression and PTSD, see Chapter 15.

Often these feelings don't come up for several months, after you've had a chance to step back from the intensity of parenting a newborn and consider how your birth went. Sometimes you won't experience grief, anxiety, or panic until your next pregnancy, when all your feelings and fears suddenly come to the surface. Traumatic births also make you more likely to experience postpartum depression.

Jealousy and Resentment

If you've had a traumatic birth, it may be difficult for you to hear about other women's birth experiences. You may be jealous of women who've had easy or uneventful labors and births, or angry at your partner for not being able to help you. Some women even find that they're subconsciously angry at their babies for being "responsible" for the trauma. Even if these feelings aren't rational, they are normal.

Working Through It

If you have negative feelings about your birth experience, it's important that you allow yourself to work through them. Write in a journal about your feelings, tell your birth story to an empathetic and nonjudgmental person, and allow yourself time to grieve. If you find that your feelings are interfering with your ability to care for your baby or yourself, seek professional help from your midwife, doctor, or therapist.

L. Essential

Sharing your birth story with others can help you work through negative feelings and come to a place of peace and acceptance. Ask your midwife, OB-GYN, or childbirth educator if she knows of any support groups for people who've had traumatic birth experiences.

You may want to read the section on emotional healing in Chapter 5, since moms who had unwanted c-sections often have similar emotional reactions as mothers who had otherwise traumatic birth experiences.

If Your Baby Has Special Needs

If your baby was born with physical or mental challenges, it's normal to feel a range of emotions like sadness, anger, guilt, and resentment. If you knew of your baby's condition before he was born, you may have had some time to process the knowledge and line up support. But if you found out at or after birth, you may be reeling with shock and anguish.

Your Friends and Family

Not being sure whether to offer sympathy or congratulations, some friends—and even hospital staff—may say nothing at all, which can leave you feeling abandoned and alone. Don't be surprised if you get as many messages of sympathy as you do of congratulations. It can be difficult when people don't know what to say to you and aren't sure if they should acknowledge your baby's birth with congratulations. If they ask you what you need, be specific: do you need someone to listen to you vent, a person to feed and water your dog while you're in the hospital, or somebody to just offer congratulations and honor your role as a mother? When people aren't sure what to do, give them some concrete ways they can help you.

Your Grief Process

It's a good idea to talk to a grief counselor when you're dealing with the knowledge that your baby is mentally or physically handicapped. In order for you to accept the child you have, you must first mourn the loss of the child you thought you'd have. Expect to go through the stages of mourning. As hard as it may seem to believe, things will get better with time.

Information and Resources

If your baby has a life-threatening or severe handicap, you're going to need a lot of support not just from your loved ones, but also from experts who can treat her. Knowledge is power; stay informed about your baby's condition, and make sure any literature you read has been published recently, since treatments and prognoses can change from year to year. You may find that your child's condition is not as devastating as you would have thought from reading literature published five or ten years ago.

Postpartum Care after a Loss

Some women must recover from childbirth after losing the baby they were carrying to stillbirth or death in the early newborn period.

Some mothers give their babies up for adoption at birth. Either situation can bring with it a confusing period of physical recovery as your body adjusts to not having a baby to care for.

If Your Baby Has Died

It's normal to experience grief, anger, and even rage after the loss of a baby you have carried. Here are things some mothers who have lost babies at or soon after birth sometimes find helpful:

- If possible, hold your baby, preferably in private. You may treasure that memory later.
- If you have access to the placenta you and your baby shared, you can take it home and bury it somewhere in your yard or another special place. This can give you a private place at home to remember your baby.
- Take a picture of your baby, or of you or your partner holding your baby. When you're feeling up to it, you can create a scrapbook of memories from your pregnancy, birth, and any time you might have had with your baby while she was alive or after she died.
- Keep items that can help you remember your baby—her hospital bracelet, a onesie, booties, etc.

Seek Out Support

Many mothers who have lost their babies find it very helpful to find others who've been through similar heartbreaks. Visit *www.honoredbabies.org* for a list of resources, support lists and groups, and a place to express your feelings by submitting an essay or poem about your baby. If you lost one or more multiple babies, you may want to visit the Center for Loss in Multiple Birth: *www.climb-support.org*. Also consider seeking grief counseling or attending a local group for bereaved parents.

Your Emotions

Responses to the loss of a baby can vary from turning quietly inward to crying and screaming in the shower. You may feel guilty or wonder what you could have done differently that would have let your baby live. Many mothers who lose their babies find themselves angry with God, their caregivers, or their partners. An intense emotional response to as huge a loss as a baby's death is normal, but if you start to feel hopeless or are unable to care for yourself or other children, tell your care provider or consult a therapist. If you feel like your family would be better off without you, or begin thinking about or considering suicide, call a suicide prevention hotline immediately: 1-800-273-TALK.

Your Partner

Be aware, too, that you and your partner may grieve very differently and you may have a hard time understanding one another's mourning process. Counseling may help the two of you communicate and work through your grief together. You may also want to consider getting counseling when you are considering getting pregnant again, since future pregnancies may be a very anxious time for you.

If Your Baby Was Adopted

If you've given your baby up for adoption, you may be feeling a huge range of emotions from sadness and anger to regret, and from guilt to relief. Some mothers who've given up their babies for adoption try to disconnect from the fact that they were ever pregnant, but your body won't let you forget—your milk will still come in, you'll be sore and weak, and it will take some time to recover. Allow yourself to experience the feelings that come up, and seek out support from other mothers who've given their babies up for adoption. Some good resources on the Web include *www.openadoptionsupport.com* and *www.lifemothers.com*.

Stopping Milk Production

When a woman's baby has died or been given up for adoption, the arrival of her milk on day three or so postpartum can act as a cruel reminder of what she has lost. To help your milk dry up, wear a snug-fitting bra or bind your breasts with elastic bandages (not too tightly) in the days after giving birth. You can place cabbage leaves with the veins lightly crushed inside your bra to help relieve engorgement. Replace the leaves when they wilt or become wet. Ice or cold packs and Tylenol or Motrin may also help with swelling and pain.

Remember, even though your baby couldn't come home with you, you are still a mother. You have given birth to a baby, and your body is creating the hormones that go along with motherhood. Be gentle with yourself and allow plenty of time for rest and relaxation as you recover, emotionally and physically, from your birth and loss.

CHAPTER 20

Going Back to Work

AT SOME POINT, many new mothers head back to work, whether they'll be returning to the office full-time, taking on a new job with more flexible hours, or returning to a modified version of their old job. If you'll be going back to work when your baby is still small, you may be feeling a range of emotions from sadness and guilt to excitement and relief. Balancing work and caring for a baby can be challenging, but with some planning and creativity, you and your baby can thrive.

Maternity Leave

The standard maternity leave offered by tradition and most short-term disability insurance policies, which you may be eligible for as a postpartum woman, is six weeks, though the Family and Medical Leave Act (FMLA) entitles qualified employees to thirteen weeks of unpaid maternity leave. When you were pregnant, six weeks may have sounded like plenty of time off, but now that your baby is here, it may not seem like nearly enough.

It may take a full six weeks to establish a good milk supply, and it will take at least that long to recover physically from childbirth. You may be just starting to feel like you've got a handle on this parenting thing by the sixth week—and aren't quite ready to deal with pumping milk, finding child care, leaving your baby, and heading to an office every day. Before you drag out your breast pump and pantyhose, consider whether you're really ready to head back to the office.

⌁ Essential

If you plan to use short-term disability benefits to cover your maternity leave, you'll want to meet with your human resources department before your baby is born to fill out paperwork and get the process started. Short-term disability pay is generally based on a predetermined percentage of your income.

Emotional Considerations

Recent research indicates that mothers who take at least three months off of work after giving birth are significantly less likely to suffer from the postpartum blues. Even taking a couple of extra weeks beyond the norm can help protect you from depressive symptoms. Also, you may just not feel ready to be separated from your baby yet. Mothers and babies are biologically programmed not to want to be separated, and this is especially intense early on.

Physical Considerations

Even if you're past the six-week mark, your body hasn't necessarily gone back to its prepregnancy condition yet. Your hormones are still fluctuating, your body is still returning to its prepregnancy shape, and you are likely operating on less sleep than you're used to. If you're breastfeeding, you need at least six weeks to establish your milk supply, which can be very difficult if you don't have constant access to your baby.

Getting a Longer Break

If you can afford it, you may want to ask for more time off or negotiate a gradual return to the workplace. If money is an issue, you may be able to patch together a longer paid maternity leave by using sick days or vacation days.

If you don't have any extra time off to use, be upfront with your employer: you love and value your job, but you just didn't realize that you wouldn't be quite feeling up to returning to work at six weeks postpartum. You may be surprised by how willing your boss is to work with you—many companies pride themselves on being family-friendly, and they may recognize that if they don't make it possible for you to focus on both your kids and your career, you may end up leaving.

 Alert

For a variety of reasons, many women have no choice but to return to work by the sixth week, or sometimes even sooner. If you're back at work before your sixth week postpartum, sit as much as possible, don't lift anything too heavy, and don't strain yourself. If your usual job is physically demanding, your employer may be required by law to give you new duties until you're fully recovered from birth.

Flexible Solutions

Though your employer may want to accommodate your needs, the logistics of making it all work may present some obstacles. It may be helpful to come to the discussion ready to offer possible solutions. This could include:

- A temporary part-time schedule, gradually adding more and more hours as you and your baby acclimate to the new situation. It may help ease your employer's mind if you plan out exactly how many hours you'll be working each week until you're full-time again.
- A job-share situation, where you split your job with another worker (maybe another new mother).
- Asking about doing some of your work at home. More and more companies are allowing employees the option of

telecommuting—working from a remote location like the home—for some or all of their working hours. You could offer to work in the office in the mornings and at home in the afternoons. Or, you could work in the office certain days of the week, and from home on the remaining days.

Reassure your boss by demonstrating exactly when you'll be able to attend to each of your job functions or make suggestions for delegating certain tasks. If your employer feels that the two of you are on the same page and working together to make your maternity leave possible for not just you but your co-workers, he or she may feel more secure in being flexible.

Consider the Costs of Working

If you want to stay home longer but think you can't afford it, make sure you're considering the costs of working. When you factor in the cost of gas, child care, work clothes, parking, and possibly extra doctor's bills—babies tend to get sick more often in day care than at home—your take-home pay may shrink considerably.

Is This the Job for You?

If your boss won't consider extending your maternity leave, you may want to consider the family friendliness of your workplace. Many situations may come up that will require an understanding employer—your baby may get sick and need to be picked up early from child care, and down the road, you may want time off for school programs and other activities. If your employer won't allow you extra maternity leave, even unpaid, how flexible can you expect them to be in the future? It's important that either you or your spouse—preferably both!—have a job that can allow for unexpected issues that pop up. If your employer isn't likely to allow you to take time off to care for a sick child in the future and your partner's employer is equally inflexible, it may be a good idea for one of you to think about looking for another job.

The Work-at-home Revolution

With the growing popularity of the Internet, creating a thriving home business has never been easier. Moms work from home in a variety of fields, providing data entry, graphic design, accounting, clerical, or medical billing services, or creating their own e-stores to sell anything from jewelry to baby diapers to soaps. Before you start a work-at-home job, make sure you clearly define your goals: Are you doing it for fun, or do you need to make a profit?

If you're replacing a paying job with a work-at-home business and need to earn a profit to help support the family financially, it's very important to look at your venture in a businesslike—and realistic—way. What kind of income do you need to make? What can you afford to spend on marketing, inventory, and other costs like shipping and Web hosting? Where will you find customers? How much can you expect customers to spend? What about returns or refunds? A business plan can help you set goals and limit unnecessary spending. Visit *www.wahm.com*, a site for work-at-home moms, for ideas, advice, and encouragement as you create and plan your business.

Breastfeeding and a Job

Contrary to what you may have heard, you can breastfeed after returning to work. It takes some planning and creativity, but many mothers successfully combine breastfeeding and a career—and it will be well worth it for you and your baby,

Should You Pump?

Some mothers are lucky enough to work close to their childcare provider, and can stop by and nurse during their lunch hours. Sometimes, Dad is home with the baby during the day and is able to bring the baby to Mom for a feeding during her lunch, or she can run home. If you have this arrangement, you may not have to worry about pumping milk as long as you aren't regularly working more than three to four hours at a time and your baby seems to be comfortable with going that long between feedings, though you may feel a little more secure if you have some pumped milk available just in case you run into a snag.

 ## Question

Are there any laws that protect my right to breastfeed and work?
Not exactly. Though all women have the right to breastfeed, most states don't require employers to support a nursing mother's efforts to pump milk for her baby. Visit *www.ncsl.org/programs/health/breast50.htm* for a list of breastfeeding laws by state.

Most full-time working mothers, however, will have to give at least some expressed breastmilk from a bottle. If your baby will be getting bottles of your milk while you're at work, you'll need to pump to keep your milk production up and maintain a steady supply of expressed milk to offer your baby each day.

What Do You Need?

Besides your breasts and your baby, there are some things that can make nursing and working a much easier match:

- **A good pump:** Hospital-grade double-action electric pumps are the best. Often these are covered by insurance. A double pump will allow you to drain both breasts at once, which means you'll get the milk in about half the time.
- **A supportive workplace:** Your employer can go a long way in making nursing possible for you by providing you with a private place and time for pumping. Talk about this with your employer, and don't feel guilty about asking for time to pump! Few people work nonstop eight- or nine-hour days. Socializing, checking e-mail, grabbing another cup of coffee—most people need, and take, mini breaks throughout the day.

- **Supportive child care:** Though feeding a baby a bottle of expressed breastmilk is just as easy as formula—maybe even easier!—your care provider will need to understand the basics of storing and using expressed milk and also be willing to work with you as you get your baby used to taking bottles. It will help immensely if your care provider is enthusiastic about your plans to feed your baby your milk.
- **A cooler or refrigerator for storing the milk:** An insulated bag with cold packs can keep your milk fresh at work. You may have gotten such a bag with your hospital going-home kit. If you have a shared refrigerator at work, you can just place your expressed milk bottles into a bag marked clearly with your name and take them with you when you go.
- **A place to store your other supplies:** You'll need a desk drawer, locker, or cubby to keep empty containers, nursing pads, and maybe a towel or extra top in case you spill or leak some milk.

Finding Time

You shouldn't let more than three hours go by without pumping, at least a little, but you don't necessarily have to have regular long pumping sessions. If you can take a short pumping break in the morning and afternoon, and one longer break during your lunch hour, that can also work. Stimulating your breasts frequently is more important than the length of time you spend pumping.

If your boss is concerned that your need to pump will keep you from finishing all your work, you can offer to come in a little bit early or leave a little late to make up for the time you'll spend pumping, or, once you get good at it, even use pumping time for work that doesn't require you to use your hands (for example, reading over documents). You may also want to point out to your boss that since babies fed breastmilk get sick less often than formula-fed babies, breastfeeding can actually help cut down on the number of personal days you'll have to take to care for a sick baby.

Finding a Place

If you have your own office at work, you can simply close the door and hang a sign that asks visitors to come back later. If you don't, you'll need to find a reasonably private area with an electrical outlet. Maybe there is a conference room that sits unused for part of the day. Or, if you know of another nursing mom in your office, ask her how she handles pumping—maybe a sympathetic co-worker will lend you her office. Some working moms even pump in the car, using a cigarette-lighter adapter. Of course, it's best if you can find a comfortable, quiet pumping station, but many resourceful moms are able to figure out ways to pump against the odds.

 Fact

No doubt about it, formula feeding is expensive—over $1,000 a year in formula alone, and up to $2,500 per year for specialty formulas. But that's not the only money you'll save: since breastfed babies get sick less often, your medical bills will be lower, too.

If Your Workplace Is Unsupportive

If you can't pump at all while at work, try pumping extra milk while you're at home and giving it to your child-care provider the next day. Try to time your feedings so that you're nursing your baby just before you leave for work and again as soon as you get home.

If you have a hard time keeping your milk supply up, you can still breastfeed. Your body will adjust your milk supply to meet demand, so you may not produce much milk during your work hours, but you can still nurse in the evening and at night. Though some babies will become frustrated at a drop in supply, many babies switch back and forth between nursing in the evenings and all night and taking bottles of formula (and, once they're older, solid foods) during the day.

Pumping Enough Milk

Some pumps, particularly cheap battery-operated on manual pumps, don't do as good a job at stimulating your milk-letdown reflex and removing milk from your breasts as the hospital-grade electric pumps do. While some handheld pumps can work great for pumping the occasional bottle, they usually aren't efficient enough to help a working mom keep up her milk supply.

If you're tense, it will be that much harder to get your milk to let down while you're pumping. Make your pumping station as cozy and comfortable as possible. In order to coax your milk into letting down, you can massage your breasts or put a warm compress on them. Relax, and try either looking at a picture of your baby or thinking about your baby to stimulate your breasts to start producing milk.

You may need to pump more often, or try pumping right after a feeding or on the opposite side during a feeding, to build up a stockpile of milk. If you are trying all this and still aren't expressing enough milk to feed your baby while you're at work, consult a lactation consultant or La Leche League volunteer for help. They can help troubleshoot and offer suggestions for pumping more effectively or increasing your milk supply.

Ľ Essential

Don't worry if you don't get a lot of milk the first few times you pump. Learning to use a breast pump efficiently requires practice and patience. After a while, you will be able to "train" your body to respond to the pump, and you'll be able to collect more milk faster.

Label containers of breastmilk before you put them in the freezer or fridge. Breastmilk can be stored at room temperature for up to ten hours, in the refrigerator for up to eight days, in a refrigerator freezer for up to two weeks, and in a self-defrosting freezer with a separate door for up to six months.

Once a baby has drunk from a bottle, bacteria can enter the milk and cause it to go bad. Therefore, once your baby is done with her bottle, you must dump any unused milk.

You can freeze milk in ice cube trays and move them to a storage bag when frozen. Each cube will be about an ounce.

Introducing the Bottle

One of the trickiest parts of breastfeeding and working can be getting your baby to accept a bottle. You don't want to introduce bottles too early because your baby may get confused switching back and forth between your nipple and the bottle nipple. But wait too long, and your baby may reject the bottle.

Many experts suggest three to four weeks as a good time to introduce a bottle of expressed milk to your baby. Some babies take readily to a bottle of pumped milk, but others aren't quite as enthusiastic.

You may want to try letting somebody else give the bottle, possibly without you in the room. Your baby has begun to associate you with nursing, and may not be inclined to accept a substitute from you with the real thing so close. You can also try offering the bottle when your baby isn't very hungry, since hunger may make her frantic and less likely to accept the bottle. But if you wait until she's completely full, she may not have much incentive to try the bottle. You may have to try a few different times to find the right balance. If your baby still won't go for it, try these tips:

- Sleep with a hand towel or cloth diaper under your shirt, and then wrap the bottle in it before it's offered to the baby. Your smell will be on the cloth, which can coax some babies to accept the bottle.
- Experiment with bottle temperatures. Some babies may want the bottle to be the same temperature as milk from the source, while others may prefer it cool or lukewarm. You may also want to heat the nipple by running it under warm water.

- Try different feeding positions. Some babies will reject a bottle when being held in the cradle hold, as it reminds them of nursing. The caregiver can try holding the baby facing out.
- There are a variety of bottle shapes and nipples available. Some babies prefer rubber, while others like clear silicone nipples. Some babies may like a wider nipple, while others prefer a longer one. You can also try the Breastbottle, a warm silicone bottle shaped like a breast. Visit ✐*www.adiri.com* to learn more details about it.
- Remain calm, and talk to your baby in a reassuring way. If you're anxious, your baby will pick up on that and may refuse the bottle.
- Get a little breastmilk onto the nipple, then tickle your baby's lips with it. When your baby tastes the familiar milk, she may pull the nipple into her own mouth.

Dealing with Guilt

Many moms feel conflicted when it comes to returning to work. You may love your job and be relieved to be going back to a familiar place where your efforts and talents are appreciated, but also may feel guilty about leaving your baby in someone else's care so that you can work. Most new mothers feel a very strong urge to be with their babies, and it can be very difficult to put that feeling aside so that you can focus on your job during the day.

Essential

Finding good child care can be daunting if you don't know where to look. Ask for referrals from friends or your midwife or doctor. Colleges and universities often offer high-quality child-care programs as part of their child-development department, or they may keep a list of students looking for babysitting jobs.

Finding a child-care situation you feel good about is one way to help ease this transition. You have many options, from an in-home nanny to a home day care or large center. Take your time with this decision, and follow what your instincts are telling you about the people who you're considering putting in charge of your baby. Some mothers and fathers work opposite shifts while their baby is very small to avoid having to use outside child care. Dads often benefit from this arrangement, since they get an opportunity to bond with the baby while you're working. You could also save a lot of money. One potential drawback is that you won't see each other as much, and your relationship may need extra attention. Don't forget to consider family as possible caretakers—siblings, aunts, uncles, and grandparents may be willing and available. Try your mom's groups—sometimes another mom is interested in providing child care. Maybe you could even trade off if your schedules allow. Whatever child-care situation you choose, be flexible and open to the idea of changing things if they don't work out.

Making Work Work

When you get back to your job, it may feel like a bit of a shock to your system. Here you are, back in a familiar place with familiar faces all around you, and yet everything is different. You may find, to your delight, that everything ran like clockwork while you were gone. Of course, the opposite is also a possibility: Your co-workers simply dumped everything on your desk for weeks, figuring you'd return one day and put it all back in order.

Stay Connected While You're Away

Since the last thing you need is to be shocked by weeks or months of accumulated work when you return to the office, it's smart to retain a connection to work and your colleagues while you're away. Keeping in touch with your bosses and colleagues via e-mail, or a few visits to the office while on break can help you communicate your needs and make sure your former duties are being handled effectively while you're gone. Don't feel pressured to step in and take care of every little problem that comes up, but being available to assist and answer questions now and then can make your transition back to the office easier.

Essential

The time you had off was just that—time off. You shouldn't have to work double-time now to make up for the weeks you were gone. If work has been piling up since you left, ask for temporary help to get up to speed.

Set Up a System

When you first go back to work, take some time to put together a time-management and organization system that works for you. If you weren't very organized before you had your baby, you may see now how important a good system is to keeping on top of the many demands you will face at once now that you have a career and a child.

And while it's important to have an organized system for handling work responsibilities, you should also have a plan in place should your baby need you during the workday. What will you do if your baby is sick or your nanny goes on vacation? Do you have a backup plan for child care—a friend, relative, or service that provides in-home care for sick kids? Maybe there's somebody at work whom you can trust to take over if you have to miss a day. Figuring this out ahead of time can make you feel less anxious.

Stay Connected to Your Baby, Too

Keep a photo of your baby on your desk, and don't be shy about calling your child-care provider to check in on him during the day. Some day-care centers even allow you to check in on your baby using Web-cam services that allow parents to view their children by visiting a Web site. The site is password protected, making it a safe and fun way to see what your baby's up to throughout the day.

Leave Work at Work

Once you're home, leave work behind and focus on your family. A special routine in the evening can help both you and your baby feel better about your separation during the day. Some working moms find that holding their babies close in the evening and sleeping with or near them at night can help them to re-create the important connection that is temporarily broken during the workday.

Take It Slowly

Allow yourself a gentle re-entry. Your first day back at work will probably be emotional, and you may find yourself crying at your desk. Allow yourself a few short workdays to ease back in to the workplace, and spend the first few days just re-acclimating yourself to your job.

Also, even if you were a "yes" employee before having your baby, now is a great time to learn to say "no." Now that you're balancing work and a baby, you'll probably feel tapped out a lot of the time. Don't take on any extra obligations unless they give you back more energy and joy than they take away.

Finally, keep an open mind and flexibility about your work situation. You always have the option to change your work schedule, find new child-care arrangements, or even quit your job if things aren't working out. Take things one day at a time, and make the decisions that feel best for you and your family now, regardless of what well-meaning friends and co-workers might have to say about it.

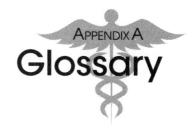

Glossary

birth plan

A document to give to the people and professionals involved in your birth experience, outlining your wishes and requests.

bonding

The process where you and your baby become emotionally attached to one another.

co-sleeping

The practice of sharing a bed with one's baby. It is sometimes called the "family bed" or "sleep-sharing."

diastasis

A separation of the abdominal muscles that can occur during pregnancy.

doula

A professional caretaker and advocate for a mother's wishes during birth. Doulas may also provide support and care to women during the postpartum period.

engorgement

Enlarged, hardened breast tissue caused by the initial arrival of milk in the breasts, or when the breasts produce more milk than is removed.

epidural

An anesthetic commonly given to women in labor. It is administered through a catheter in the back and delivers medication to the spinal cord to reduce or eliminate sensation in the lower half of the body.

episiotomy

An incision made through layers of tissue and muscle in the perineum to widen the vaginal opening during childbirth.

foremilk

The milk your breasts produce first during a feeding. Foremilk is usually thin, and looks bluish or watery.

hindmilk
The creamier, fattier milk that your baby receives near the end of the feeding.

hormonal contraception
Medications or devices that help prevent pregnancy through the use of hormones.

hormones
Substances, produced by a gland or organ, that enter the bloodstream and affect other parts and processes in your body.

incontinence
The inability to control the leakage of urine, and more rarely feces, that sometimes occurs after giving birth.

lochia
The mixture of blood, tissue, and fluids that flows from the vagina after giving birth.

mastitis
An infection of the breast, often caused by engorgement, which can cause chills; fever; and a red, hard, painful area of the breast.

maternity leave
The time mothers take off from their jobs immediately before or after the birth of a baby. A father's time off is called paternity leave.

milk ducts
The passages in the breast that carry milk to the nipples.

oxytocin
This hormone helps the uterus to shrink to its normal size after childbirth, and stimulates the breasts to produce milk.

NICU
Stands for newborn intensive care unit, the area in many hospitals that cares for babies who are born early or who are sick at birth.

perineum
The area of tissue and muscle between the vagina and the anus.

placenta
The organ that nourished and provided oxygen to your baby during pregnancy. Delivery of the placenta is called the third stage of labor.

postpartum mood disorder
This label encompasses a variety of mood disorders, including postpartum depression and anxiety, that can occur in the weeks and months after giving birth.

thrush
A yeast infection that can infect a mother's nipple or the inside of a baby's mouth.

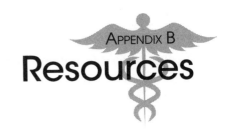

Resources

Organizations

DONA International

DONA International is a professional organization with more than 5,500 birth and postpartum doula members. The organization serves mothers and families by providing access to information and research about doulas, childbirth, and the postpartum experience. There's even a searchable database of doulas on the Web site.
✍ *www.dona.org*

International Lactation Consultant Association (ILCA)

The ILCA is the professional association for international board-certified lactation consultants (IBCLCs) and other health-care professionals who care for breastfeeding families. You can find a wealth of information, as well as a directory of lactation consultants, on the Web site.
✍ *www.ilca.org*

La Leche League International

La Leche League is an international volunteer organization that offers information and support to breastfeeding mothers. The Web site will connect you to discussion forums, podcasts, and other resources to help you get your breastfeeding questions answered.
✍ *www.lalecheleague.org*

Postpartum Support International

Postpartum Support International is an organization aimed at increasing awareness among public and professional communities about the emotional changes that women experience during pregnancy and the postpartum period.

✎ *www.postpartum.net*

Books

After the Baby's Birth by Robin Lim
A holistic guide to making a healthy spiritual, emotional, and physical transition to motherhood.

The Baby Book: Everything You Need to Know About Your Baby from Birth to Age Two by Dr. William Sears
Written by an experienced father and pediatrician, this baby-care book helps parents trust their instincts and care for their babies with compassion and sound information.

Beyond the Blues: A Guide to Understanding and Treating Prenatal and Postpartum Depression by Shoshana S. Bennett, Ph.D. and Pec Indman, Ed.D., M.F.T.
Packed with information and advice to help women and their families recognize and manage prenatal and postpartum depression.

The Everything® Breastfeeding Book by Suzanne Fredregill
Advice and easy-to-follow information to have a successful and enjoyable breastfeeding experience.

The Everything® Mother's First Year Book by Robin Elise Weiss
A comprehensive guide to the first twelve months of motherhood and caring for baby.

The Nursing Mother's Companion by Kathleen Huggins
A complete and thorough guide to breastfeeding, including troubleshooting and information on work and pumping.

*Taking Charge of Your Fertility: The Definitive Guide
to Natural Birth Control, Pregnancy Achievement,
and Reproductive Health* by Toni Weschler
This book is very comprehensive and informative, and the corresponding Internet community (✍*www.tcoyf.com*) makes it easier for women to figure out trickier situations—like breastfeeding or Polycystic Ovarian Syndrome (PCOS).

Web Sites

About Single Parents
About.com's guide to single parents, Jennifer Wolf, guides you through both the joys and trials of single parenthood. The Web site has lots of great resources, including a discussion forum where you can chat with other single parents.
http://singleparents.about.com

BirthPartners.com
This Web site has a directory of all different kinds of natural birth partners, including postpartum doulas. You can also find links to articles, product information, and other resources.
✍*www.birthpartners.com*

The Cleaning Service Directory
This nationwide directory of housecleaning services offers resources for everything from carpet cleaning to window washing so you can get the help you need during postpartum.
✍*www.house-cleaning-services.com*

Making Lemonade
This is an online single-parent network providing advice, resources, and support to single parents.
✍*www.makinglemonade.com*

The MOMS Club

This is a great support group for at-home moms.
✍*www.momsclub.org*

Moms Rising

Interested in activism? Check out this online grassroots movement dedicated to motherhood and family issues.
✍*www.momsrising.org*

Mothers & More

This nonprofit organization is dedicated to supporting women who are sequencing—taking some time off of work, reducing their hours, changing their jobs, or otherwise taking the mommy track.
✍*www.mothersandmore.org*

A Nanny on the Net

No matter what state you live in, this nationwide agency can help you find a nanny who fits your needs. Their Web site has resources like applications and FAQs.
✍*www.anannyonthenet.com*

Nannyville

Nannyville is an online directory that helps parents find nannies. You can see a free preview of their current nanny applicants before you register to become a member.
✍*www.nannyville.com*

The Online PPD Support Group

This Web site offers a number of helpful resources, including discussion forums, recommendations of books and publications, true stories from families that have experienced postpartum depression, and more.
✍*www.ppdsupportpage.com*

The Postpartum Stress Center

The Postpartum Stress Center specializes in the diagnosis and treatment of prenatal and postpartum depression and anxiety disorders. The PPSC also offers a full range of general counseling services to individuals and couples seeking support.

www.postpartumstress.com

Index

The Everything® Health Guide Series

Supportive advice. Real answers.

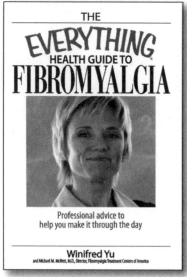

Trade Paperback
ISBN: 1-59337-586-7
$14.95 ($19.95 CAN)

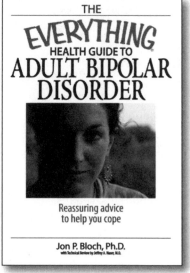

Trade Paperback
ISBN: 1-59337-585-9
$14.95 ($19.95 CAN)

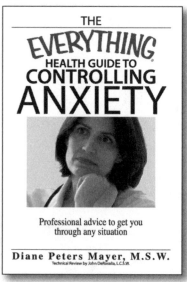

Trade Paperback
ISBN: 1-59337-429-1
$14.95 ($19.95 CAN)